COUPLE SEXUAL AWARENESS

Also available from Carroll & Graf:

Sexual Awareness by Barry & Emily McCarthy
Male Sexual Awareness by Barry McCarthy
Female Sexual Awareness by Barry & Emily McCarthy

OUPLE SEXUAL AWARENESS
Building Sexual Happiness
Barry and Emily McCarthy

Carroll & Graf Publishers, Inc.
New York

First Carroll & Graf edition 1990
Second printing 1991
Carroll & Graf Publishers, Inc
260 Fifth Avenue
New York, NY 10001

        Library of Congress Cataloging-in-Publication Data

McCarthy, B. (Barry)
    Couple sexual awareness : building sexual happiness /
Barry and Emily McCarthy. — 1st Carroll & Graf ed.
        p.   cm.
    Includes bibliographical references.
    ISBN 0-88184-592-2 : $9.95
    1. Sex in marriage.   I. McCarthy, Emily J.   II. Title.
HQ31.M37   1990
613.9'6—dc20
                                                    90-1685
                                                        CIP

Manufactured in the United States of America

CONTENTS

I. Enhancement

II. Dealing with Problems

1
IS THERE SEX AFTER MARRIAGE?

We know that sex comes naturally, that there are clear rules governing successful marriages, that being happy with your marriage is the norm, and that if you love each other and communicate everything will be fine. Right? Wrong! Such unrealistic expectations are a major source of frustration and unhappiness in American marriages. Many couples lack awareness and understanding of the complex processes involved in both marriage and marital sex.

This book is directed to those of you who want a satisfying, stable marriage as well as fulfilling marital sexuality. You will learn concepts and techniques to help change your attitudes about respect, trust, emotional intimacy, and sexual expression. We will present guidelines to improve marital communication and sexual satisfaction. Instead of dictating one right way to be happy and successful, we believe each couple needs to develop their own marital and sexual style.

Sexuality is not the most important factor, but it is integral to marriage. Sexual expression serves as a shared pleasure, a means of tension reduction, and most importantly increases intimacy. When sex goes well in a marriage it is about 15 to 20 percent—it serves to energize the marital bond. When sex is problematic, it can drain positive feelings and be a major impairment. In marriages where sex is dysfunctional it can become 50 to 75 percent of the marriage.

We urge couples to avoid the happily-ever-after approach to marriage. We emphasize the importance of "couple time" and the necessity to allocate psychological energy to ensure satisfaction in the relationship. Marriage is an active, ongoing process, not a static state that can be taken for granted.

SEXUALITY AND MARRIAGE

Cultural, parental, and peer pressure to marry abound. Over 90 percent of people do marry. Among the more than 40 percent who divorce, the great majority remarry. Marriage is the most popular voluntary institution in America. But often marital intimacy—like a freshly cut rose—blooms early and then fades into habit and routine. The concept of a genuinely intimate and sexually satisfying marriage draws disbelief, guffaws, and cynical remarks from many people.

Most sex books have been directed toward the young, with discussions of premarital sex, "meaningful relationships," and finding the "right" person to marry. It would appear that sexuality begins at sixteen and ends at twenty-five, its prime purpose to get the person safely—without disease, an unwanted pregnancy, or a hurtful relationship—settled into a marriage by the age of twenty-one. The image is of a movie in which the couple marries, has totally satisfying intercourse with simultaneous orgasm, and, with the assumption that they live happily ever after, "The End" flashes on the screen. Unfortunately—or rather, fortunately—life, sex, and marriage are more real and complex than that.

The focus of this book is on the reality and complexity of your marital and sexual bond. Sex does not belong to youth and the newly married. You are a sexual person from the day you are born until the day you die. Sexual experiences during marriage constitute the major portion of most people's sexual lives, yet this area has received surprisingly little scientific or public attention. It is a subject hidden behind self-defeating attitudes.

WHO WE ARE AND WHY WE WROTE THIS BOOK

In the process of reviewing research, doing clinical work with couples, conducting sexual enhancement workshops, teaching human sexuality, and thinking about our own marriage, we have come to believe that several concepts are central. One is the importance of setting aside couple time and valuing intimacy; another is being aware of sensuality, which is the basis of sexual responsivity, and the central role of pleasurable, nondemand touching; the importance of multiple stimulation and the freedom to let go and enjoy arousal and orgasm; and the crucial need to reduce performance anxiety and replace unrealistic expectations with a more flexible, pleasure-oriented, broader-based view of sexuality in marriage. The main purpose of this book is to offer concepts and techniques to help the couple develop a more intimate sexual relationship that will add to marital satisfaction and stability.

We write from the dual perspective of clinical practice in marital and sex therapy, and our personal involvement in the subject matter. Barry is forty-six and Emily forty-four. We have been married twenty-three years and have three children—Mark, Kara, and Paul. This is the fourth book we've written together, and integrates our views about the role of marriage and sexuality. Throughout it we will be offering case material as well as observations from our life—not as the ''right'' methods for you, but as concrete illustrations of how real couples change and negotiate transitions in their marriage.

POSITIVE GUIDELINES

Our premise is that your marital and sexual relationship will be more satisfying if based on solid information. Awareness and attitude change are necessary, but not sufficient. The couple must change their manner of relating. Expectations must be reassessed, communication skills improved, and it is important to understand and cope with the challenges of aging, to adopt a less performance-oriented, more pleasure-oriented view of sex, and to increase the frequency and variety of affectional, sensual, and sexual interactions. As attitudes and behavior change, feelings of closeness and intimacy grow.

We do *not* believe there is only one way. In fact, we feel just the opposite. Each individual and each couple has a unique set of experiences, attitudes, values, preferences, feelings, and life situations. Each couple needs to develop the marital and sexual style that satisfies their needs and desires.

It is amazing to realize that couples who do well and are knowledgeable in other areas can be naïve about their marital relationship and sexuality. We see couples who are financial wizards and know a great deal about "the good life," but whose marital lives are essentially zero. Americans value marriage as an institution, but few are taught how to communicate feelings, build intimacy, make sexual requests, increase marital commitment, and enjoy intimate sexual experiences. The challenge is to integrate these guidelines and skills so you can have a more intimate and secure marriage.

WHAT IS YOUR MARITAL AND SEXUAL STYLE?

What do we mean by a marital and sexual style? By the time they've been married two years, a couple has established a pattern of roles and behaviors—for example, who gets up to make the coffee, or who chooses the kind of music they listen to. They have established a style of intimate communication that may be functional, but more often is not. The couple may talk over coffee, but their conversation will be about sports, neighborhood events, finances, chores, or children's activities rather than a sharing of personal perceptions and feelings.

Until the last twenty years, little research had been done to increase our scientific knowledge about adult sexuality. Even the so-called experts—psychologists, physicians, ministers, marriage counselors, and teachers—were minimally helpful, their advice based on theoretical notions or common myths. With the breakthrough research of Masters and Johnson and other behavioral scientists, our understanding of marital and sexual functioning has increased dramatically. The more information you have, the better is your position to make reasoned and productive decisions.

Our culture is heavily influenced by notions of romantic love. Couples strongly believe that love is enough. Loving feelings are necessary, but certainly not sufficient for a good marriage. Romantic love, which idealizes the partner and relationship, needs to be replaced by a broad-based, mature, and stable sense of emotional intimacy. This means acceptance of the real person and the strengths and weaknesses of the relationship. Intimacy allows you to deal with problems and failures as well as loving feelings and sexual highs. It energizes you to deal with the real and complex issues present in an ongoing marriage.

Our behavior is influenced by the models, especially parental models, that we have observed. Most couples haven't learned to be a communicative, sexually comfortable couple from their parents, who were influenced by their own parents and the lack of information and antisexual attitudes of the culture at that time. Parents are viewed as nonsexual by their children. They are seen as parents only, rather than as individuals and as a sexual, married couple. An informal study conducted in Barry's human sexual behavior course found that only one in four college students could imagine their parents having intercourse and only one in twelve could imagine their grandparents being sexual.

In addition to the absence of a parental model for marital sexuality, most couples lack a good model for marital communication. Children usually see parents talking over family/child issues or practical problems. Anger is either irrational, destructive, or violent, or there is no expression of angry feelings. Seldom do children witness their parents expressing emotional support for each other or in constructive disagreement. And heaven forbid that parents touch or kiss where the children might see them. The best way to learn a behavior is through modeling. Few couples have experienced good models of marital communication or even seen an affectionate couple. We will present positive models of how to become emotionally intimate and sexually comfortable.

SPECIFIC COUPLE STRATEGIES AND TECHNIQUES

An excellent way to learn and grow is by employing specific change strategies and techniques. The strategy that most influences our marital relationship is "private, couple time." This is time we set aside for the two of us, without children—to talk about individual and couple feelings and issues rather than practical matters. It is a time that could be associated with sex—for instance, twenty minutes after intercourse—but need not be. A couple might sit over a drink, go for a walk to talk over personal concerns, share something they are happy and excited about, or discuss how they have been getting along the past week. We encourage setting aside at least one period a week for private, couple time. Some couples do this three or four times a week. This time does not *just* happen, it's *planned* to happen. It needs to be recognized as an important priority, planned into and valued in your busy schedule.

One of the benefits of marital therapy is that it provides a structured time to talk as a couple. When marital therapy ends, Barry encourages couples to preserve this time since it's already built into their schedules. But instead of an office visit and a fee they go to lunch, take a walk, or meet at home and make love. Emily believes a major communication aid in our marriage are our walks two or three times a week during which we share feelings and perceptions, deal with issues, make plans, or just enjoy companionship and the beauty of nature.

Once a month, or every other month, try to set aside a day that is primarily for yourselves as a couple. Keeping a relationship fresh, close, and enjoyable is a constant process of sharing experiences, communicating feelings, and giving yourself time and permission to be intimate. It is necessary to have time away from jobs, children, the phone, and friends. This allows you to experiment with sexual techniques, learn a new sport or hobby, or just be together in a relaxed atmosphere. One of the most prevalent and self-defeating social myths is that marriages do not need time or attention after the initial adjustment period. Your marital bond needs time, psychological energy, and continued attention if it is to remain vital and satisfying. If businessmen put as little time and energy into their businesses as most couples put into their marital relationship, we would have a bankrupt country. With so little attention, it's amazing marriages do as well as they do!

In an intimate, satisfying marriage there are four things a couple needs to be able to do:

1. Communicate with and support each other.
2. Be able to deal with bad feelings in constructive ways.
3. Laugh, enjoy each other, and share interests.
4. Have a satisfying sexual relationship.

The more comfortable and skilled the couple are in these areas, the more intimate and satisfying their marriage will be. These are not inborn traits, nor do they naturally develop, even if a loving relationship exists. They are learned skills that require awareness and effort. Like any skill from playing tennis to cooking, once learned it needs to be refined and practiced.

Don't allow your marital and sexual relationship to become routine and stagnant. Marriage can be a continual process of changing and growing. As the poet/philosopher Kahlil Gibran said, "A love that is not always growing is dying." One key to successful marriage is a commitment to integrate individual and couple changes. The marital relationship is a *process*. It is changing not only at twenty-five, but also at forty-five, and just as much at seventy-five. You never stop learning and growing as a person, as a couple, and in your sexuality.

COMMUNICATION AND EMOTIONAL SUPPORT

When we speak of communication skills and supporting each other emotionally, we are referring to a series of component skills. These are:

1. Empathic listening for content and feelings being expressed.
2. "Checking out," especially for intentions.
3. Empathic responding.
4. Use of "I" communications.
5. Making requests instead of demands.
6. "Going my way" skills of negotiation.
7. Reaching agreements both can live with.

The first and foremost skill is listening to your spouse in an empathic manner, understanding both the content *and* feelings being expressed. Because of different socialization males attend to content and ignore feelings, whereas females focus on feelings and attend less to content. This is a major cause of the communication gap couples complain about. Take time to listen to your spouse, trying to "take the role of the other," to understand the issue from your spouse's viewpoint. When you assume you are right and your spouse is wrong, you fail to listen to perceptions and feelings. Instead, you are waiting for the spouse to finish so you can make your point. To be a good communicator, you must first be an empathic listener.

The second component skill is "checking out" to be sure you understand what was said, the intention, your spouse's feelings, and what is being requested of you. Reacting defensively, as if attacked, or as if demands had been made, puts the couple in competition rather than on the same team and trying to communicate. If you feel pressured or hurt by your spouse's comments, checking it out allows you to determine whether that was the intent, or if you misunderstood the message, or if it was expressed in an unclear way. It is particularly important to check out your partner's intentions—is she trying to be helpful and make a positive point or is she feeling angry and undercutting? One way to check out is to say, "I feel put down by your comment; did you mean it as a put-down?" Checking out before responding makes it more likely that your response will be constructive rather than defensive or a counterattack.

A third component skill is empathic responding, which means that you respond with your feelings and requests, keeping in mind your partner's perceptions and feelings. This is very different from disparaging the other person, giving "yes, but" responses, or counterattacking. Share your perceptions and feelings and express them within the context of working together. Strive to communicate in a respectful and responsive manner. The goal of empathic responding is for your partner to know he was heard and to respond with your feelings and perceptions.

A fourth component skill involves using "I" communications. This means saying "I want to go the movies today; are you up for it?'' ''I feel sensuous right now and would love to get a chest rub; are you interested?'' ''I really think we need to talk about our finances,'' or ''I want to go out to dinner tonight.'' Be clear, direct, and straightforward with your feelings and what you want. Take responsibility for yourself and be your own agent rather than reacting to your partner or how you think she wants you to be. This is very different from a couple communication pattern of ''What do you want to do?'' ''I guess you want to have sex,'' or ''I don't care; how do you want to handle it?'' ''I'' communications are honest. With them you take responsibility for your feelings and behavior. They involve taking risks and making you more vulnerable to being disappointed, but it's worth it.

Make requests, not demands. The fifth component skill is learning to make clear, assertive requests. This replaces communication which is either passive and indirect or is aggressively demanding. A major difference between a request and a demand is that the request gives the partner a choice. You might not get precisely what you requested. You choose to work with your partner rather than intimidate or coerce him. A demand puts pressure on the person to give you what you want when you want it or there will be consequences. It is the difference between saying, ''I would like you to stroke my penis slowly'' and ''You better turn me on by playing with me, or you won't get any tonight.'' Sexual demands cause sexual dysfunction and resentful feelings; sexual requests result in pleasurable sex and feelings of emotional intimacy.

Going my way? The sixth component skill is learning to generate alternatives and to set the stage for negotiating agreements. When two people with their own needs and preferences relate intimately, they have to be open to negotiation. A crucial negotiation technique is to replace a simple ''No'' with ''No, I am not willing to give you a thirty-minute back rub, but I would like to sit and snuggle for a few minutes.'' Instead of ''No, I have a headache,'' you could say, ''I have a headache, and would like a neck rub. Let's see how I feel; we might stop there, have intercourse, or I could stimulate you.'' In place of saying no and cutting off communication, offer an alternative that is acceptable to you. Your partner can decide if he is open to engaging in the alternate activity. People mistakenly feel that if they cannot have what they want when and how they want it, they are not loved. The reality is that you do not usually get things exactly your way. Couples fall into the power struggle trap: "my" way against "your" way rather than a couple style of communicating and negotiating—"our" way.

The seventh component skill is negotiating worthwhile agreements. Agreements are very different from compromises. Always compromising is a common couple trap. In compromises, neither person gets what he wants; both go along with a compromise neither enjoys. For example, if one wants to go to a French restaurant and the other wants Chinese food, they compromise on standard American fare, which neither wanted nor do they enjoy. At a minimum, a couple needs to reach agreements both can live with. Ideally, they would negotiate an agreement in which each gets something and feels better about the relationship because of it

Negotiation, where you clearly state your feelings and wants, listen to your partner's, and try to reach an agreement in which both of you get at least some of your needs met, is preferable to the process of compromise where you do something neutral so that neither feels he or she has lost. In this brand of compromise, you both lose! Making requests and considering alternatives adds to the sense of caring. For example, the man might want fellatio and the woman might want a sexual massage with body lotion. They compromise by having sex with the woman on top, which is not what either wanted. But in a sexual agreement, the woman might receive a sexual massage with lotion and then reciprocate with a sexual massage which includes fellatio and integrates multiple stimulation during intercourse with a quiet and close afterplay. You can reach agreements that are satisfying to each person, and in so doing, you become a more intimate couple.

EXPRESSING NEGATIVE
FEELINGS IN CONSTRUCTIVE WAYS

Many couples believe that arguing is the opposite of intimacy. That's a self-defeating myth. Intimate couples *can* and *do* have bad feelings. It's important to be able to express them. Some couples brag that they never fight. Such relationships are built on an unrealistic premise that presents a strong risk of explosion, resulting in feelings of hurt and betrayal. Learning to express feelings in an honest and constructive manner is a vital skill. It isn't easy, but it's worthwhile.

For a relationship to continue growing, both partners need to feel they can be honest, open, and vulnerable. This includes feelings of love, caring, and respect as well as feelings of hurt, anger, and disappointment. You can say, "I am feeling angry with our poor financial situation." This is very different from, "You are a failure, you'll never learn to handle money." Each person needs to acknowledge feelings, to describe the situation in an objective way with the intention of problem solving, and to avoid blaming the spouse.

Learning to argue well does not mean that you fight over each matter, or let your spouse know immediately about each feeling, and it certainly doesn't mean physical intimidation. These behaviors are inappropriate and aggressive, just as the couple who never fight is overinhibited and frightened of feelings.

Learning to argue constructively includes three component skills:

1. Being able to express feelings.
2. Expressing feelings in a nondestructive way, without "hitting below the belt."
3. Requesting a specific change in your spouse's attitude or behavior that will alleviate your feelings and the problem situation. The intention is to engage in constructive problem solving.

The first component skill—clearly stating feelings—means saying, "I am hurt and angry when you come home three hours late and don't call me" instead of "I hate you, you're an inconsiderate bastard.'' It means saying specifically what you are feeling and what is causing you to feel that way. It does not mean calling your partner names, blaming or attacking, or saying she always does it and is hopeless. It involves communicating your feelings and trying to solve the problem, not getting your way or making him feel guilty. Good arguing skills include staying on the specific issue and feeling instead of dredging up past feelings or incidents. Stay with here and now issues and feelings. Don't refight battles of the past and throw in old incidents, the proverbial ''kitchen sink'' fights.

A second component skill involves arguing in nondestructive ways. It means saying, ''I feel hurt, confused, and angry when you don't show me the consideration to call'' instead of ''You're irresponsible and manipulative just like your mother.'' One of the best things about an intimate relationship is that you feel safe, trustful, and accepted for the person you are. You can reveal your vulnerabilities, the sad or bad moments of your life, fears and inadequacies, without dreading that they will be used against you. In a destructive fight, that is just what happens. Your vulnerabilities and weaknesses are used to attack you, and you feel betrayed and angry. In retaliation, the spouse ''goes for the jugular.'' The argument degenerates into a destructive power struggle or, in the colloquial, ''a pissing match.'' The couple is no longer trying to achieve anything, each spouse is fighting not to lose. The worst example of this kind of degenerative fighting style is demonstrated in the movie *Who's Afraid of Virginia Woolf?* Couple fights can turn into physical abuse, especially if one or both has been drinking.

Focus on your feelings rather than castigating your spouse. Be honest in owning your feelings rather than blaming them on the partner. If, during an argument, one hits below the belt, the offended spouse should not immediately counterattack but say ''I felt you just gave a low blow; did you really mean to do it?'' Most of the time, the spouse was simply caught in the heat of the argument. When made aware by your comment, the spouse backs off from his hurtful attack. If the spouse will not back down, or is maliciously being hurtful, be aware that this argument can only be destructive and that you would do better to leave the fight situation. After a cooling-off period, when both are willing to argue constructively rather than engaging in an increasingly more out-of-control fight, you can return to the issue.

The best time to air feelings and argue is when you have time and privacy to talk and problem solve. An important guideline is not to have arguments after midnight—nothing constructive happens between then and six in the morning—or when one or both people have been drinking. In terms of sexual issues, have sexual arguments when you're clothed and not in bed. Sexual arguments when you're nude and lying down make you too vulnerable to destructive comments.

Couples use arguments as a means of emotional catharsis, getting gripes off their chests. You feel better for a while, but frustrations and anger build because the situation has not changed. It is important to express feelings rather than build resentments. But just expressing the feeling is not enough!

The third component is to clearly and directly request a change that will alter the problem situation and alleviate your bad feelings. It is important to state your feeling clearly: "I feel hurt because you did not pay attention to me last night." "I'm disappointed that after you said you'd try the side-by-side intercourse position, you stopped when it was awkward." "I am frustrated when we make plans to solve financial problems and don't follow through." "I am disappointed that you forgot to attend our daughter's recital when you promised you'd be there." It is just as important to make a specific request for change: "When I say we need couple time, I want us to find a time we can talk or to go dinner and enjoy an evening out." "From now on, each week we will go over the family budget." "You need to apologize to Sue yourself rather than my doing it for you. Why don't you do something special with her next week?" Statements like "You have to change your attitude." "You will never change," or "You do not care" are nonproductive and will not bring the changes you want. Taking a problem-solving rather than blaming approach, making specific requests for change, and following through on behavior change plans has the greatest likelihood of alleviating distressing feelings and situations. The more pervasive and chronic the problem, the more detailed a plan you'll need. This includes a more active monitoring process and the establishment of a series of smaller goals to facilitate gradual change.

Of the skills and attitudes we write about, the constructive expression of bad feelings is the hardest to integrate into our marriage. Our arguments involve tears and hurt feelings, at least on occasion. We have a commitment, and a strong one, to avoid insulting each other or making the partner feel guilty. Our major difficulty is waiting too long to discuss the feeling because we don't want to complain about a spouse we love, one who is attentive and considerate in most ways. We find that once the issue is aired and an agreement made, it was worthwhile to express the feelings and deal with the problem. We have some chronic problem areas, especially regarding finances, which we are unable to satisfactorily resolve. On occasion, we need to air feelings about the problem so that frustrations and resentments do not build.

LAUGHTER AND SHARING

Coules are not naturally compatible. They need to evolve an enjoyable, satisfying style of being together, to learn to laugh, enjoy activities, and share interests. Having two or three activities which both people genuinely enjoy is the base of couple interaction. This could include playing tennis, going to movies, playing cards or board games, eating ethnic foods, being active in a community group, listening to jazz, dancing, decorating your house, going camping, gardening, participating in a church discussion group, golfing, reading poetry, going to car races, traveling, or entertaining. Not all activities can or should be joint. Having nonshared interests and activities is good for an individual and can be beneficial to the marriage. The husband having a night out bowling with male friends or taking a class and the wife having a bridge game with female friends or being involved in a woman's group are ways of establishing your individuality. Each couple needs to decide on a healthy balance of individual and couple activities.

Couples who shared experiences when first married may find they've grown apart and are involved in other activities and separate friends. Individual interests, activities, and friends are fine, but not at the expense of shared interests. Activities you'd done fifteen years ago might no longer be enjoyable, although you still do them out of habit. It is possible to revitalize old interests like going to plays you enjoy and discussing them afterward. Be open to developing new interests, such as taking Chinese cooking lessons or square dancing. These interests might include practical tasks—you could learn to hang wallpaper or finish furniture. It's important that at least one activity involve being playful, whether it's playing bridge, taking hikes, playing racquet ball, going to musicals, or visiting exhibits. It's important to share pleasurable activities.

Being able to laugh and accept idiosyncrasies and foibles is necessary; each of us has our weaknesses and irritating behaviors. Accept that some things just do not work the way you hoped rather than reacting with anger and disappointment. For instance, if the couple tries making a new dessert for a dinner party and it comes out absolutely awful, it's better to laugh it off rather than trying to pretend everything is fine and embarrassing the guests and yourselves. The ability to laugh at yourselves is especially important in the sex area. Even couples who are very satisfied sexually find that in 5 to 10 percent of their sexual experiences, things do not go well. The sex might be mediocre, boring, or a downright "bomb." Overreacting and becoming dejected or frustrated can be replaced with a healthy acceptance that even the best of couples have mediocre or poor sexual experiences. The couple who stop the sexual activity, laugh, and say that tonight is just not our night for sex is a couple who will continue to have a good sex life.

A SATISFYING SEXUAL RELATIONSHIP

This leads us to our final skill area—building and maintaining a satisfying sexual relationship. Sex is *not* the central ingredient in marriage, but sexuality is an integral component of the marital bond. Sex serves as a reinforcer and energizer. When the couple's sex life is poor, it depresses and negates other aspects of the marriage. A lack of regular, fulfilling experiences creates a void. Sexual problems drain a marriage of positive feelings. There are times in every marriage when things are dull, stressful, or unsatisfactory. During those times, it is valuable to share satisfying interactions, including sexual ones, to help you through.

There are three elements to a satisfying sexual relationship:

1. Feelings of intimacy and desire.
2. Comfort with sexual communication, nondemand pleasuring, and making sexual requests.
3. Functional and pleasurable sexual expression (including multiple stimulation, intercourse, and orgasm).

Sex is a natural physiological function, like breathing and eating, but the components of satisfying sexual functioning are learned as a result of experience and feedback. We have devoted an entire book, *Sexual Awareness:Sharing Sexual Pleasure,* to a discussion of specific exercises to help a couple learn to communicate and function better. The principal skills are the ability to enjoy sensuous, nondemand pleasuring and to make sexual requests, guiding your spouse in how to touch and stimulate you; learning to accept and follow your partner's guidance; being open to a range of sensual and sexual experiences; the use of multiple stimulation, including fantasizing, to build arousal; saying no and requesting alternative pleasuring scenarios; multiple stimulation before and during intercourse; using focused, rapid, rhythmic thrusting as you approach orgasm; letting go and being orgasmic; having pleasant afterplay scenarios; and learning how to laugh or shrug off unsatisfactory sexual experiences. Most important is to put pleasure and intimacy into your sexual life rather than seeing sex as a goal-oriented performance. The essence of sexuality is giving and receiving pleasure within the context of an emotionally intimate relationship.

One of the most prevalent sexual myths is that marital sex naturally becomes less frequent and enjoyable because you have learned all you can and tried everything there is to try. No matter how often you have sex, you can never experience all the variations and complexities of being with someone you love. In a truly creative, intimate relationship your own as well as your spouse's desires, feelings, and awareness continue to evolve. As you age, you have different feelings, perceptions, and responses. The couple who fall into a dull, stereotyped sexual relationship have no one to blame but themselves. Sexuality can and should be a positive force in marriage. Focus less on performance and quantity and enjoy a more pleasurable, intimate, and higher quality sexual relationship. Youthful emphasis on frequency and performance are replaced by middle-years emphasis on quality, pleasure, and satisfaction.

Some people, including our editor, wondered why we chose to focus this book primarily on sexual intimacy as compared to other aspects of marriage. Sex in marriage has traditionally been ignored and viewed as an unglamorous topic although it does play an integral, energizing role in the marital bond. When being sexual, the couple are most open and intimate, which is one of the special experiences that makes being married worthwhile. With the growing awareness that divorce has more repercussions on individuals, children, and society than originally believed, and with the fear of AIDS, couples are more motivated to make their marriages work. Sexuality is a vital component in satisfying and stable marriages.

The greatest need for marriages, including our own, is the consistent expenditure of time and psychological energy. Sexuality is much more than intercourse and orgasm. Sexuality includes the walks you take, affection inside and outside the bedroom, nondemand pleasuring, discussing intimate feelings while clothed, sharing touch and feelings before and after intercourse, and times when, verbally or physically, genitally or nongenitally, you express intimate feelings. Sexual expression can and does energize the marital bond and promotes intimacy, satisfaction, and stability.

THE PLAN OF THIS BOOK

This book is *not* intended to be do-it-yourself marital or sex therapy. Our intent is to increase understanding of marital and sexual functioning by presenting guidelines on improving communication, arguing in constructive ways, negotiating change agreements, learning to laugh and enjoy couple activities, and engaging in sexual experiences that are pleasurable and satisfying. For couples having difficulties—probably 50 percent of marriages—we present suggestions to deal with issues and problems.

Chapters examine the marital bond, sexual variations, sexuality education for children, the transition to being a couple again, and preparing to be a sexual couple after sixty. Additionally, chapters explore problem areas such as sexual dysfunction, extramarital affairs, dealing with illness, second marriages, and the more mundane stresses of day-to-day marital living. A critical concept is the husband-wife bond as the primary relationship in a family.

We focus on these four themes—communication and support, expressing negative feelings constructively, laughing and enjoying each other, and having a satisfying sexual relationship—throughout the book. This manuscript is not like a novel in which you read each chapter in turn. Although there are continuities among chapters, each is self-contained and has its own theme. Read those that are of immediate import to you. Some chapters could be read alone, others with your spouse; you might even read aloud to each other. However, reading is not enough—you need to discuss the concepts and guidelines and try to integrate them into your life and marriage. This book could be read for concepts, information, and attitude changes, but it will have maximum value if it serves to help you develop strategies and specific techniques to improve your relationship.

Sexuality is an integral component of the marital bond. A satisfying sexual relationship promotes shared pleasure, tension reduction, intimacy, and energizes the bond. Marriage requires continued psychological time and energy. Contrary to popular myth, couples report increased sexual satisfaction over time.

Older couples are less athletic sexual performers but are more intimate, high-quality lovers.

Some couples become aware of dissatisfaction or problems as a result of discussing issues raised in this book. Marital and sex therapy can be valuable in helping them work through communication difficulties and untangling problem areas. Some have bad reactions to the idea of counseling or therapy, seeing it as a sign of personal weakness, craziness, or that their marriage is in big trouble. On the contrary, seeking professional help is a sign of strength. You are admitting problems, agreeing to work together to alleviate sources of concern, and choosing to consult a professional who can facilitate your communication and problem solving. We have included an appendix on how to choose a marital or sex therapist.

Awareness that each person and each couple is unique is the basis of our approach. We hope the concepts and guidelines presented will encourage you to attend to your relationship and help you develop your special marital and sexual couple style.

2
THE MARITAL BOND—RESPECT, TRUST, AND INTIMACY

Throughout this book we emphasize sexuality as positive and integral to your marital relationship, but *not* as the most important factor. This chapter will focus on core dimensions of the marital bond. Sex will hardly be mentioned.

In most books about marriage, communication is given prime billing—communicating feelings, needs, perceptions, and values. Many experts, if not most, believe empathic, clear, and direct communication guarantees a successful marriage. According to these experts, communication is the principal element in marriage.

We certainly believe in and stress the importance of communication, but do not view it as the prime element of a successful marriage. In our conceptualization the essential components of the marital bond are respect, trust, and intimacy. Emotional intimacy will be emphasized in this chapter, although both emotional and sexual intimacy are vital for marital satisfaction.

Some couples play a communication game—pretending to communicate about a problem when, in fact, one partner has already determined how he or she wants it resolved and uses power to implement the decision. An example might clarify this.

Carol and Tim. Carol and Tim had a marriage that was characterized by friends as open, sharing, and communicative. They would talk about their feelings about every decision. However, when the chips were down, the decision made was almost always what Tim desired. Their explanation was that although Tim listened to and understood Carol's feelings and concerns, it was only logical to do it his way since he had the heavier schedule, made more money, and could not change his appointments. Besides, they rationalized, Carol was overly emotional and sensitive.

A prime basis for the marital bond is respect for each other, trust that your partner has your best interests in mind and will not subvert agreements or intentionally undercut you, and a sense of openness, vulnerability, and emotional intimacy. Within this framework, the principles of open, clear, and direct communication are of great value. These same communication techniques in the context of a nontrusting relationship with a gross power imbalance are destructive. The communication process is a sham in a relationship like Carol and Tim's. For communication guidelines to be worthwhile there needs to be equity in the distribution of power, self-respect, respect for your partner, and a trusting relationship. Otherwise, communication techniques can be used in a manipulative or coercive manner.

RESPECT, TRUST, AND INTIMACY

These concepts are interrelated, but we will examine each separately and then discuss integrating them into your couple bond.

Respect. Respecting your spouse and accepting his or her strengths and weaknesses is the basis for a mature, intimate relationship. Knowing, understanding, and accepting the partner, which is the basis of respect, clashes with the media stereotype of romantic love. Respect emanates from a clear view of your spouse. It is not based on an emotional, rose-tinted perspective that ignores behavior or personality traits that are problematic. Romantic love idealizes the partner, respect entails knowing the partner's positive and negative traits while still respecting and loving him.

Respecting your spouse does not mean you have to agree with everything she does, nor does it mean that there will be no changes in behavior. A marriage works best when based on a positive influence model of change.

Respect includes not demeaning your spouse, especially in front of children or friends. It encompasses working with your spouse as a supporter, as opposed to being an antagonist or competitor. When she is experiencing a serious problem at work or with the children, or is phobic or depressed, the spouse can be empathic and supportive, not blaming or condescending. Be aware of and emphasize your partner's strengths and avoid dwelling on his failings. People love us for our strengths; our spouse loves and respects us for our strengths and weaknesses. For example, Barry acts like a fish out of water when it comes to repairing articles around the house and Emily nearly hyperventilates if she has to entertain more than two people. We acknowledge problem areas without losing respect for each other. When there is a difficulty that needs to be dealt with and changed—Barry not monitoring his diabetes or Emily ignoring financial responsibilities—the issue is confronted, but in a problem-focused, nonpunitive way. We try to avoid engaging in finger-pointing. Maintaining an equitable balance of power in the marriage is crucial to personal respect and respect for the spouse.

Trust. Talk of respect turns many couples off. They fear that love and romance have been taken out of the relationship and replaced by a realistic, functional partnership with little emotion. We believe respect is a necessary, but certainly not sufficient, basis for a satisfying and secure marriage. Trust and intimacy are vital and add special feelings.

Trust integrates pragmatic and emotional components in marriage. Marriage is a functional relationship between two people, but to be satisfying it must be more than that. Trust that your partner cares about you, and has concern for your best interests, is crucial. Trust involves caring about your partner as well as his caring about you. A trusting relationship means believing that your spouse would not intentionally hurt you or subvert your needs.

Trust in your spouse is the emotional basis of a satisfying marriage. Couples under stress or experiencing a crisis will successfully make it through as long as the sense of trust in their "coupleness" remains intact. Once this trust has been breached, it is difficult, although not impossible, to regain. All couples experience stress, bad feelings, anger, disappointment, and conflict of needs. If a sense of trust is maintained, they can deal with these and emerge a stronger couple, having learned from and survived the stressful situation.

Intimacy. Emotional intimacy is the special component that energizes and nurtures the marital bond. A chief ingredient in intimacy is freely and comfortably self-disclosing feelings, thoughts, and perceptions. This means revealing positive and negative feelings. Our preferred model of marriage is one in which the couple view each other as intimate friends whose secrets, perceptions, feelings, hopes, and problems are shared. Some couples prefer having more emotional distance in their marriage, which is fine as long as it is agreeable to both people. A new myth is that you can never have too much emotional intimacy. You need to retain your individuality; intimacy does not mean total emeshment and giving up your sense of self. Trouble arises when one demands more intimacy and the other demands more distance. The couple needs to establish a mutual comfort with their degree of emotional and sexual intimacy.

Emotional intimacy includes developing a comfortable way to be with each other. Some couples enjoy talking about feelings and aspirations. Other couples do best when talking is combined with an activity like walking, playing board games, going to dinner, working on a household chore, attending a concert, or playing golf. Being a couple includes, but is certainly not limited to, discussion of intimate feelings. Integrating talking and touching is an important ingredient in intimacy.

Being there for each other in difficult and sad times, as well as sharing moments of joy and success, is integral to couple intimacy. To paraphrase Kahlil Gibran, there are many people you can laugh with but you especially value people you can cry with. Special elements of intimacy are celebrating happy moments as well as acknowledging that you have survived intact painful or traumatic experiences. Being there for tough times makes the intimacy bond stronger.

Tonia and Roger. Tonia and Roger recently completed a couples' communication training workshop. It was a high-quality, professionally-organized group where they learned effective techniques to listen and respond empathically—eye contact, nonverbal attending, verbal acknowledgement, and reflecting feelings. Yet they continued to fight and marital dissatisfaction was increasing. After a consultation with their minister, they were referred to Barry for marital therapy.

After three assessment sessions it was clear that intimacy and communication were not the core problems for Tonia and Roger. The therapeutic focus was on their marital agreements and how they decided—or more to the point didn't decide—who did what in the relationship.

Tonia worked three-quarter time as a secretary. She had almost full reponsibility for Jill, their eleven-year-old daughter, as well as full responsibility for the house. Couple and social activities were organized by Tonia. Roger was quite unhappy with his job as an inspector for the buildings department, and this job unhappiness dominated his life. He complained incessantly about money and his work. Roger spent Sunday afternoons drinking beer and watching sports on TV.

Roger and Tonia loved each other and communicated about a variety of issues, including parenting their daughter, friendships with other couples, and relationships with in-laws. But love is not enough to sustain a marriage. Couples have to maintain respect for each other and be able to talk about and solve problems.

The topic they studiously avoided was that Tonia did not respect the way Roger handled his job frustration. She understood and empathized with his feelings, but did not like how he was dealing with them, and felt that he was acting like a macho teenager. When the issue finally was confronted, Roger did not react defensively. He was not proud of his passivity about the job problem. He maintained that since the situation was as it was, and since his job brought in a great deal more money than Tonia's, she had no right to hassle him about how he spent his time and handled frustrations. Feeling a surge of power and assertiveness, Tonia began making demands of Roger, who felt that she was pushing him around and did in turn, become defensive and resentful. This could easily have degenerated into a bitter power struggle that would have threatened their basic sense of trust. Marriages work best when they are based on a positive influence model which promotes respect and trust and from that basis addresses and resolves problems. It is preferable to confront a difficult issue in a respectful and problem-solving manner.

A further complication, which intrudes on many marriages, is that each spouse talks to same-sex friends who support their viewpoint. Roger's male friends assured him that women hassled their husbands and wanted them to be "good little boys." The only way to deal with women was to show them who was boss and ignore them. Tonia's friends told her men were unreliable and wanted to be "playboys." The way to make your point was to threaten to leave or to withhold sex. With friends like this, you don't need enemies. Unfortunately, too often, friends and family members take sides and make judgments that exacerbate marital difficulties and sabotage the communication/problem-solving process.

Barry encouraged Tonia to use her communication skills to make clear and direct requests, and to avoid making demands, issuing ultimatums, or disparaging Roger. Roger in turn was urged to listen to her requests and take a hard, objective look at his attitudes and behavior. His job frustrations were real, but he allowed them to dominate everything. He resolved to resume control of his life, and made a commitment either to change his job within the department or, failing that, to seek another job. Realistically, it could take at least six months to engineer a satisfactory job change. During this period he resolved not to use his job frustration as a way to avoid marital and parental involvement. Specifically, Roger agreed to limit his drinking/sporting with male friends to once a week. If something special was coming up, he would consult Tonia before making plans with friends.

Roger had ignored his responsibilities to Tonia, Jill, and the house. He wanted to resume those responsibilities, and Tonia was surprised by her reluctance to give them up even though, intellectually, this was what she wanted. This is not unusual—it's hard to give up power and prerogatives, whether you're a woman or a man.

Once the power balance, the sense of mutual respect and trust returned, the same communication techniques that had been unhelpful three months before became worthwhile for Roger and Tonia. They experienced a renewed sense of emotional and sexual intimacy. Most important, they had a commitment to problem solving and reaching mutually acceptable agreements.

Power. The women's movement has made us acutely aware of power issues in relationships. The traditional model, in which the man was supposed to be in control of household, financial, and family decisions because he earned more money, with the wife as handmaiden in charge of cleaning, cooking, and children, was never valid. Men believed money equaled power, and since traditionally they were breadwinners, they did not have to share in less pleasant tasks such as housecleaning, changing diapers, and driving children to activities. There is too much emphasis in our culture that money equals power, but that *definitely should not* be so in a marriage.

A joke among therapists is that the most difficult people to treat are two lawyers overconcerned with protecting their bargaining positions and not showing any weaknesses. Techniques that may be effective and appropriate for the business world are harmful in intimate relationships. Power plays and intimidation do not work in marriage. They might serve to get what you want in a specific situation, but in the long run they're costly for the relationship. The resentment that builds and the desire to retaliate are destructive to the marital bond. Power manipulation allows you to win a battle, but you lose the war for a successful marriage.

Couples report greater satisfaction when there is an equitable sharing of power. Each spouse will have areas in which he or she takes more initiative and is dominant. Because a spouse accepts the partner's initiatives in a given area does not mean he is powerless. Power is not something that is shared fifty-fifty on each issue. Equal power in all areas is an unrealistic expectation and an unworkable model. Feeling comfortable with your sense of power and being aware of the spouse's power facilitates an equitable balance which allows respect, trust, and intimacy—including sexual expression—to grow.

COMMUNICATION

Good communication techniques facilitate marital functioning. In the first chapter we discussed the following communication skills:

1. Emphatic listening for both content and feelings.
2. "Checking out," especially for intentions.
3. Empathic responding.
4. Use of "I" communications.
5. Use of requests instead of demands.
6. "Going my way" skill of negotiation.
7. Reaching agreements both can live with.

We won't repeat ourselves, but will focus on communication exercises. Marital communication is an ongoing process based on assumptions that each person's needs and feelings matter, that you trust your spouse is negotiating in good faith rather than engaging in a power play or placating you, and that an agreement, not empty promises, will result in behavioral followthrough. An example of that process gone awry will illustrate the importance of communication.

Jenny and Tom. Jenny and Tom had been married twenty-two years and were able to work out most aspects of their marital relationship, except for one persistent problem area. At issue was the amount of time Jenny spent on the phone talking to friends. This had been a sore point for over twenty years. It was such a conflict that they avoided talking about it, since talking always ended in a replay of the same shouting, accusatory fight. The problem wouldn't go away. When Tom came home in a bad mood or when he wanted to talk to Jenny and found her on the phone, he'd make a snide comment, and a cold war began that could last for days.

In trying to communicate about a chronic, difficult problem, a crucial guideline is to approach it anew with a commitment to stay focused on the present and refuse to refight old fights. One suggestion is to use an outside person—someone you both like, trust, and who is willing to do it—as an objective resource to keep you on task. Tom and Jenny had the discussion with the help of a mutual friend whose profession was labor relations negotiator.

The format gave each time to speak. The partner's role was to empathically listen for both feelings and content, in a respectful and caring manner, undistracted by worries about what to say, or trying to make a point. Then the roles were reversed. They took their time and went through the process conscientiously instead of rushing ahead to reach an agreement.

Jenny wanted Tom to understand that she enjoyed talking with friends. This was not a reflection on him, although she also wanted Tom to listen to her, especially when she talked about events of the day and things she was worrying about. Tom felt rejected, hurt, and angry that she cared more for her friends and the telephone than for him. Both agreed that this was a serious problem. Each felt that the other did not understand and should change.

Once they could see the emotional and content issues more clearly and did not get off task by refighting battles and bringing up old hurts, it was possible to negotiate an agreement. Jenny agreed to talk with her friends no more than half an hour when Tom was in the house. If she was on the phone when Tom came in, she'd break off the conversation in five minutes. If need be, she could call the person back. Tom agreed to spend more time listening to Jenny's feelings and not to perceive her talking on the phone as a personal rejection. In making this agreement, they felt validated even though neither got exactly what he wanted. They agreed to treat a problem incident as a lapse and not as a negation of the entire agreement or a reason to start the argument/cold war again. This is crucial—even when you communicate clearly and come to an agreement, it does not mean the issue/problem will never again rear its ugly head. Problems and irritations occur in the most solid marriages and when the couple has the best of intentions. Hopefully, when the issue comes up again, you're better prepared to handle it in a problem-solving manner. The best technique is simply to reinstate the previous agreement and act accordingly.

The marital communication process is ongoing. You can't rest on your laurels. There are no perfect people and no perfect marriages. Don't blithely say, "We communicate about in-laws," or "We communicate about money," and leave it at that. Especially as parents age, new issues arise concerning in-laws, and in our age of competition and economic change you have to communicate regularly about money matters. To facilitate the communication process, we suggest the following exercises. These are techniques we have used in our marriage and found of value.

COMMUNICATION EXERCISE ONE: Sharing

Once a week for a month, set aside at least one hour with privacy and no interference. Turn off the TV and put on the telephone answering machine, or take the phone off the hook. You have only one agenda—to share something about yourself and discuss feelings. No problem solving, no financial or parenting decisions, no talk about neighborhood or politics—the agenda is you, your spouse, and your individual and couple perceptions and feelings. We suggest the following format:

1. State your perceptions and feelings as clearly and directly as you can, using "I" language.

2. Before your spouse responds, she repeats what she heard. Be sure the spouse understands your perceptions and feelings before moving on.

3. The spouse then states his perceptions and feelings clearly and directly, using "I" language.

4. Again, make sure the spouse's perceptions and feelings are understood.

When couples are given this task, their initial reaction is to see it as too mechanistic. The exercise has a valid focus—to force you to slow down the communication process, to really listen to your spouse's perceptions and feelings, and to respond with your own (defensiveness or counterattacking is not appropriate). Try to put yourself in the role of the other. At first this will feel awkward, but as you become more comfortable and refine your communication skills, you will be able to use these techniques with greater flexibility. It's a bit like learning tennis: at first formal and structured, but once you learn the basics, adapt it to your game—in this case, your couple communication style.

COMMUNICATION EXERCISE TWO: Sharing a secret

Set aside at least an hour of private couple time. Before your communication date, spend time alone thinking of an experience you have not shared with your spouse. The secret you choose to share need not be a bad one. It can be any experience, attitude, dream, or feeling you've not previously shared. The secret could be feelings about your first date, a fantasy or dream you've had, an embarrassing childhood experience, the first time you ever did something entirely on your own, a past event you felt humiliated by or ashamed of.

Begin by stating your motivation for sharing this secret and what you want from your spouse. The reason for sharing your intention is to reassure your spouse, as well as to remind yourself, that you are not doing this hostilely or as a way of "getting" your spouse under the guise of openness and honesty. Do you want feedback, support, suggestions, or just acceptance? Some people prefer to state their secret at the beginning, whereas others want to discuss the context, motivations, and feelings before sharing the secret. Whichever way you prefer is fine—as long as you do it.

Once shared, don't let the secret drop. Discuss your feelings, and how she feels about your secret. Stay with the feelings it evokes; don't avoid or analyze your partner's reaction as a way of diverting your focus. People who guard secrets from everyone, including spouses and best friends, run the risk of not feeling fully accepted as a person. You tell yourself that if someone knew your secret they would think less of you or reject you. You need to be able to accept yourself with all your disappointments, traumas, and embarrassments, and feel understood and respected by those close to you, especially your spouse. Don't switch to discussing your partner's secret until you've fully discussed yours. Allow a few days lapse before discussing the spouse's secret.

Once you've had the experience of sharing a secret, it is easier to discuss feelings about other sensitive areas in a more flexible, less formal manner. It might give you permission to share a more personal or difficult secret—about fears of failure or childhood abuse, for example, or having been fired, or having been personally or sexually humiliated.

COMMUNICATION EXERCISE THREE: Your parents' marriage as a model

Parents are a major influence, especially regarding what you learn about marriage from observing them and their patterns of communication. People associate therapy with the stereotype of the "shrink" who analyzes childhood feelings and discovers that the root cause of all problems is the parent. Actually, therapists no longer make childhood memories their primary focus, and we certainly do *not* recommend that you do so in your marriage. We do not agree with therapists or popular writers who engage in "mother bashing" or "father bashing." This exercise is oriented in a very different direction—to increase awareness and understanding concerning your parents and their marriage.

In discussing your parents' marriage, first highlight aspects of it that you admire and would like to incorporate into your own marriage. Then pinpoint the aspects of your parents' marriage that you view as unsuccessful or inappropriate. Consider these as psychological traps for you. These areas must be approached with careful thought and planning so that your life and marriage operate differently.

It's difficult to be objective about parents; there is a tendency to be emotional/subjective and to make either overly good or bad generalizations. Try to be as specific as possible with both strengths and weaknesses. It can be valuable to hear your spouse's perceptions of your parents' marriage, especially if the spouse is objective and specific. You do not have to agree with your spouse—after all, they're your parents—but these perceptions can broaden your perspective.

The focus is on how parental models influence your marriage. Don't throw your spouse's disclosure about his traps in his face during a fight. One of the advantages of an intimate marriage is that you can share concerns and vulnerabilities without fear of being abused or taken advantage of.

This exercise is to encourage you to spend more time and energy thinking about your marital and family life. You are an adult, responsible for your life and marriage. Accept that responsibility—don't blame your parents. This exercise can help you see them more objectively as people with their own strengths and weaknesses. Perhaps it will even help you to deal more effectively with your aging parents.

COMMUNICATION EXERCISE FOUR: Expressing negative feelings and requesting specific changes

The idea of scheduling an argument is a far cry from traditional marital advice. There are conflicts in all intimate relationships. A crucial couple strategy is to communicate hurt or angry feelings and request changes before those feelings blow up into a major, destructive fight. Most couples do not feel right about proceeding in this more rational, problem-solving manner. They see it as more natural to have unplanned, explosive, destructive fights. Expressions of hurt and frustration are necessary in a relationship; name-calling, vindictive fights are not.

One partner takes the initiative and brings up an issue she is hurt or angry about. Don't blame your partner for these feelings. They're your feelings, and you need to take responsibility for them. Use "I" language ("I feel hurt") not "you" language ("You're to blame for hurting me"). Once you've expressed those emotions, pick one issue and stay with it. Don't raise other problems. Once your partner understands your feelings and perceptions about the issue, make a clear, specific request for change. Remember, it's a request, not a demand. Your spouse can decide whether he chooses to accept your request or offer an alternative to change the situation. Be sure this issue is aired and a change negotiated before going on to the spouse's feelings and request for change.

The partner's feelings/request should be dealt with at a separate time and treated as a separate issue. This is to reduce the possiblity of counterattack on the same or a closely related issue. The purpose of stating feelings and requesting a change is not to overpower, intimidate, or embarrass your spouse. This exercise is not a competitive game with a winner and a loser. When you learn to share hurt feelings, make requests, discuss alternatives, negotiate changes, and reach mutually acceptable agreements, your marriage is the winner.

The process of taking responsibility for and stating your feelings without blaming, demanding, or threatening and of staying with one issue until its resolution are vital skills.

COMMUNICATION EXERCISE FIVE: Acknowledging strengths and accepting compliments

For many couples, this is the most difficult exercise. We say we want more compliments, that we want people to give us pats on the back. We are disappointed and even bitter when we don't receive a "thank you" or a kiss to acknowledge the good and caring things we do. Yet we have a hard time genuinely listening to and accepting compliments, especially from the most intimate person—our spouse. We suggest that the wife go first because in our culture women have been discouraged from being complimentary about themselves and acknowledging their strengths. Little girls are told to be quiet and proper, not verbal and vain.

Set a timer for three minutes. You have three minutes to talk about positive aspects of yourself and your strengths, with your spouse listening attentively. Say only positive things without qualifications. Give yourself permission to say, "I am proud of the way I planned and built the patio," not "I did okay but it wasn't as good as the Jones's professional job." State the attributes you respect and like about yourself. Look at your spouse as you speak, without being embarrassed or apologetic for "bragging on yourself." Three minutes is a short period of time, but some people feel it's an eternity when the task is self-acknowledgment. You owe yourself at least three minutes to be positive.

When you've completed the self-acknowledgments, your spouse has three minutes to say things about you that he values. He can reinforce what you've said, but it's especially worthwhile if he chooses strengths and positive attributes that had not been mentioned or downplayed. Don't be afraid to mention points that seem small; the only guideline is that the feelings and statements be genuine.

You could change roles during this exercise or wait a day to reverse roles. Be as honest as possible; don't try to compete with your partner by saying more things or giving just the right compliments. After you've completed the exercise, spend time discussing how you felt about giving and receiving positive acknowledgments. It will become easier to give and receive compliments and to acknowledge the aspects of yourself and your spouse that you value.

CLOSING THOUGHTS

These five communication exercises are designed in a structured, formal manner. Your ongoing communication need not be structured or formal. We suggest that you regularly share feelings, discuss difficult issues, talk about family and in-law patterns, be able to confront bad feelings and ask for change, and give compliments and acknowledge positive attributes. Communicating comfortably permits you to feel secure and satisfied with yourself as a person and your marital relationship.

For a stable and satisfying marital bond, there needs to be a sense of equity in respect, trust, and intimacy as well as clear, comfortable, and genuine communication. As with sexual aspects of the relationship, once you've achieved this balance, you cannot rest on your laurels. You change as people and your relationship changes. Devote time and psychological energy to reinforce the marital bond.

3
NONDEMAND PLEASURING

In most people's experience the line between affection and sex is very clear. Affection is something you do with clothes on, involves kissing, hand-holding, and/or hugging, and can be done in public. Traditionally, affection was viewed as the domain of women. Sex involved nudity and its goal was intercourse and orgasm. Traditionally, sex was the domain of men, but increasingly it has been recognized that women have sexual needs and feelings. Affection and sex have been viewed as altogether different and separate activities by both women and men.

Awareness of nondemand pleasuring introduces an entirely different way of conceptualizing and experiencing affection, sensuality, and sexuality. It challenges the arbitrary distinctions of the traditional approach, and most importantly discards the view that women and men are alien in their emotional and physical need for touch. Nondemand pleasuring does away with the dichotomy between affection and sex, viewing touch as a continuum from hand-holding to intercourse. Affectionate touching can occur inside or outside the bedroom, may be initiated by men or women, can be done while clothed, semi-clothed, or nude. It meets needs of both women and men for physical and emotional closeness.

An integral component of the pleasuring continuum is the concept of sensuality. Sensuality is experienced in private, includes some degree of nudity, involves experiences like bathing or showering together, back rubs, body caresses, and slow, tender, exploratory, caring touching. Sensuality includes both nongenital and genital touching. It is pleasure-oriented, not orgasm-oriented.

Sex is more than genitals, intercourse, and orgasm. We are unequivocally in favor of both intercourse and orgasm, which are integral to sexual satisfaction. When you limit sex to intercourse you cheat yourself, your sexuality, and your marriage of a range of affectionate, sensual, and sexual experiences. Affection, sensuality, and nondemand pleasuring provide the basis for sexual satisfaction in marriage.

Couples who are open and receptive to nondemand pleasuring report more closeness and touching, and more intercourse and orgasm too. There are many ways to express intimate feelings, and many bridges to develop sexual desire. Some women avoid engaging in extended, sensual kissing unless they desire to have intercourse. If she felt free to kiss in a sensual manner, for its own sake, to elicit desire for a later time, or to see if kissing resulted in arousal, there would be more opportunities to feel sensual and sexual. The male might caress his spouse's breast or have her touch his penis with a sense of playfulness and openness that would increase the exchange of pleasure and opportunities for intercourse. If breast and penis touch is restricted only to times leading to intercourse, there will be fewer playful times and less intercourse. Nondemand pleasure, which includes affection, sensuality, and sexual touching, is integral to the relationship, not restricted to the bedroom before and after intercourse. Couples who have only two gears—the first a ritual kiss in the morning and at night and the second gear intercourse and orgasm—miss opportunities for pleasure and sexual intimacy.

Nondemand pleasuring is an excellent example of how the premarital attitudes of women and men interfere with marital sexuality. If touching is to strengthen the marital bond, the wife and husband have to overcome their adolescent misconceptions and enjoy a range of nongenital and genital pleasuring. Affec-

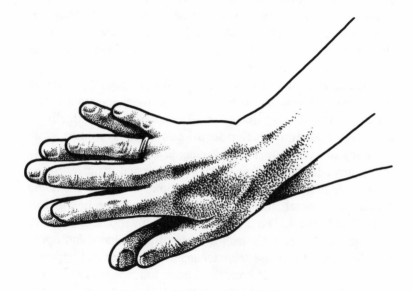

The basis of non-demand pleasuring is comfort with touching. Put your hand upon his and show him how and where you like being touched.

tion, sensuality, sexuality, and intercourse can be valued by both people.

Jan and Craig. As an adolescent Craig both loved and hated petting games. He loved the sense of adventure and conquest when he'd "get farther," but was frustrated that the woman held power and would not let him have "the real thing." He swore that once he was married he would never play those games again. Jan had a very different perception of touching and quite different experiences. She enjoyed the romanticism and sense of play that accompanied kissing and caressing. However, she felt pushed and imposed on by men wanting more breast and genital stimulation, and tired of defending herself against the accusation of being a "tease." She hated the pressure of having to say "no" and continually pushing the man away. What could have been a pleasurable experience turned into a struggle.

Jan and Craig met during their junior year in college when they were dating other people. Both were aware of an attraction, but since each was involved with someone else, they focused on developing a friendship. When they returned to school the following year, Jan learned that Craig was no longer dating the same woman. They met for a cup of coffee, and Jan remembers feeling strongly attracted and a special sensation when Craig touched her arm. As they left the café, he took her hand and they went for a walk in the woods surrounding the campus. Their first kiss was gentle, exploratory, and sensuous. If this had been a movie they would have thrown off their clothes and made wild, passionate love. Jan was ambivalent because she had a sense of loyalty to her boyfriend. Craig wanted a relationship with Jan, but worried that it would turn into a triangle and a bad scene—he'd seen that happen too often with friends. They were holding hands when they walked out of the woods. Jan promised to call Craig if she chose to pursue the relationship. After soul-searching, talking with friends, and a sad and angry confrontation with her boyfriend, she called six days later.

Senior year of college is a time of major decisions and transitions, but what Jan and Craig remember were the delicious moments of their love affair. Jan was taking birth control pills, and they began having intercourse almost immediately. Their lovemaking consisted of much more than intercourse. There was public affection, especially kissing—which Craig particularly liked—and hand-holding—which was Jan's favorite medium to express affection. They watched television or listened to tapes curled up in each other's arms. There was lots of kissing, caressing, and stroking, clothed and unclothed. The romantic love experience is special and not to be missed. Craig enjoyed touching, nongenital as well as genital. When it culminated in intercourse, which was most of the time, Craig found it particularly gratifying. He saw Jan was open emotionally and sexually, not as a woman who played games. He believed that she would be loyal, and for the first time in his life he was committed to being sexually faithful. This was the most satisfying relationship Jan had ever had. She viewed Craig, in a more idealized and romantic way than was true, as interested in emotional expression, affection, and sexuality—the perfect man.

Craig was an engineering major and through a co-op program was committed to working in another state. Jan had planned to go to graduate school, but for the sake of the relationship chose to postpone that for a year and move with him. Although she is glad she married Craig, she regretted the decision not to continue with her career plans; she did not return to graduate school until thirteen years later.

Living together is very different from dating and proved to be a difficult transition. There is the advantage of time and privacy, but you have to deal with practical and mundane matters which makes your time together less special. It is different sleeping in the same bed each night. The sense of romanticism and unpredictability is gone. This transition was harder for Jan than Craig. Jan's parents were unhappy that she was not continuing her education and displeased that she was living with a man. Jan saw her job as temporary and not particularly satisfying. She would not have chosen to live in that town. Craig was excited about his career, was developing a mentor relationship with his boss, and making friends with co-workers. Craig enjoyed the regularity and stability of their living together and the rhythm of intercourse four to five times a week. As all too often happens, the special moments and affection were taken for granted and they fell into a routine.

Touching and affection decreased, but sexuality and intercourse remained the same. This pattern occurs with both nonmarital and marital couples. It's not a conscious decision, just an easy trap to fall into. Although Jan was aware of dissatisfaction, it wasn't acute so she decided not to voice her concerns. She felt better when Craig said, "Let's get married before the end of the year since we'll have to make another move for my job."

Although many magazine articles would claim that there isn't much difference between living together and being married, that is not the reality for most couples, nor was it for Jan and Craig. Marriage is best viewed as a commitment to lead a life together and share plans, goals, values, and emotional and sexual intimacy. When Jan and Craig married it was with the hope and belief that the marriage would be satisfying and secure. They were pleased to join their lives, emotionally, financially, and practically. Jan hoped that with marriage there would be a return to affection and playfulness, but did not voice this. Unfortunately, affection continued its gradual downhill slide. It was not that Jan was dissatisfied with Craig, the marriage, or sexual intercourse, but that she missed the touching, sensuality, and special moments.

Twelve years later Jan and Craig appeared at a therapist's office. The stated problem was concern over their nine-year-old son's school underachievement. The clinician did an evaluation of the entire family, not just the boy. The recommendation was for special tutoring in reading for the son and consultation concerning what the parents could do to increase academic motivation. They were pleased with those suggestions, but were taken aback by the recommendation to seek marital therapy. The clinician felt that Jan was depressed, and that marital dissatisfaction was the cause. At first Jan felt defensive, but on reflection admitted that the assessment was correct. She was interested in discussing her concerns about the marriage with a professional. Craig was considerably more reluctant, but was persuaded by the argument that relationship problems are more likely to be successfully resolved in couples therapy than in individual therapy and that therapy could prevent a marital crisis. The child psychologist referred them to a marital therapist she highly recommended.

The assessment format was to see Jan and Craig together, then each separately, and then a couple feedback session to discuss the issues and propose a course of treatment. In Craig's individual session, he stated few concerns. The primary one was that intercourse frequency had declined to once a week, typically on Saturday night, and almost always at his initiation. He rationalized that with their busy lives and schedules this was to be expected. Jan had many more concerns and complaints. The primary one was the disappearance of the sense of specialness and affection. She enjoyed sex when they got around to it, but reported feeling emotionally distant from Craig, not connected physically, and that the marriage was item ten on his busy agenda with the first seven items involving his job.

In the feedback session, the marital therapist said he was glad they'd come at this point because in another year the marriage would have been in crisis. He emphasized to both, but especially Craig, that this was the time to reverse direction and get back on track. He made a number of observations and suggestions, the most important having to do with couple time and nondemand touching. The easy, affectionate touching they'd experienced premaritally and early in the marriage had almost disappeared. There was little public affection other than routine kisses and little cuddling or stroking except in bed on weekend nights, almost always as a prelude to intercourse.

The therapist made it clear that nondemand pleasuring was not a return to adolescent necking and petting games. It was a cooperative effort to revitalize affection and sensuality. It is a good sex education model for children to see their parents kissing, holding hands, hugging, and cuddling. It is not appropriate to be sensual or sexual in front of children (these forms of sexual expression are private acts.) Knowing their parents are loving and affectionate is reassuring for children. The therapist encouraged affectionate touching inside as well as outside the bedroom as a way of relearning that touch is critical in promoting emotional bonding. Touch is neither a signal or a demand for intercourse or orgasm-oriented sexuality.

The therapist commented on their almost total absence of sensuality. He suggested they take a bubble bath and/or a relaxing, sensual shower where they washed each other. This is something they had not done, even in their early days. The novelty made it a special experience. Craig was out of touch with his sensual needs, but did enjoy washing Jan's back and Jan toweling him dry. For Jan the sensual experiences caused a reawakening of special feelings. Although the therapist made a point to Craig that sensual experiences were not meant to be a prelude to intercourse, it was Jan who initiated intercourse following the experience. Jan felt sensuous, desirous, and aroused. Intercourse was a natural continuation of those feelings. As they discussed that experience themselves and in therapy, there were several important discoveries. Foremost was how important nondemand pleasuring was to Jan and how much she had missed it. Craig acknowledged that he'd enjoyed it and wanted this to be a part of their intimacy. He found sensuality a new experience and a worthwhile bridge between affection and sexual expression. A second discovery was how satisfying it was to engage in slow, nondemand touching and how important to reconnect emotionally and physically. Sensuality can have a strong effect on sexual desire, which was particularly striking to Jan. The therapist emphasized that although sensuality could and often does serve as an impetus for sexual expression, it is not an expectation or demand. Sensuality works best in the context of a nondemand experience which is valued in and of itself. It serves as a bridge for sexual intercourse only when one partner is desirous and the other is open and receptive to the invitation.

Jan and Craig learned that comfort with affection and sensuality is the basis of sexual desire. This is especially important for marriages of over two years duration.

NONDEMAND PLEASURING AS
A BRIDGE TO SEXUAL INTERCOURSE

Nondemand pleasuring is the single most important component in sexual intimacy. It can and does serve a number of functions, one of which is a bridge to sexual desire and intercourse. For some couples, it is their favorite way to initiate intercourse. For others, sensual experiences such as showers or baths, full-body massages and chest or back rubs, using lotion as an adjunct to touching, are a way of relaxing and a bonding experience. This can engender desire, arousal, and a transition into intercourse. Sensuality best serves as a bridge to intercourse when it is viewed as a couple process, not when one partner has a hidden agenda of wanting intercourse but is not willing to ask for it or when sex is viewed as a teasing, withholding game. The decision to proceed to intercourse is a mutual one which evolves from the sensual interaction and a desire to extend it.

Less than half of sensual experiences proceed to intercourse for the typical couple. Some couples engage in sensual experiences three to four times a week, others once a month or less. There is a positive relationship between openness to sensual experiences and frequency of intercourse. Sensuality fans the flames of desire and increases the couple's sense of comfort and connection.

Tina and Howard. It is nice to see couples who have a comfortable sense of touch. You are most likely to see this among unmarried couples in their twenties—a not very funny joke is that you can tell married from unmarried people because married couples don't hold hands or touch in public. Tina and Howard are in their early fifties and provide a powerful antidote to that perception. They enjoy being with each other, touching, and being touched. As Tina proudly says, "We come from touching families and our children touch in their marriages." What matters most are the small touches—stroking his cheek as Howard wakes up, a kiss that lingers a few seconds, Howard patting Tina on the rear in the kitchen, a hug before leaving for work, teasing stroking of a breast or penis to carry a pleasing memory during the day, a gentle kiss when arriving home rather

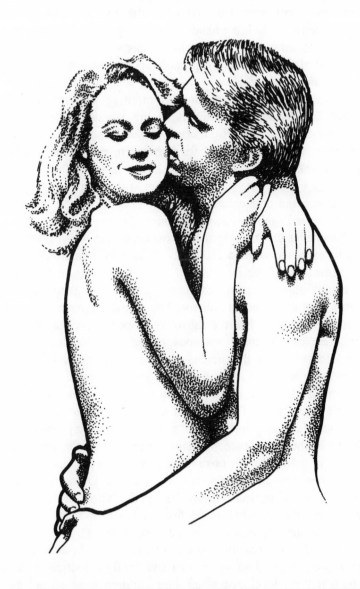

Non-demand pleasuring is the single most important component in sexual intimacy. Sensuality can be enjoyed for itself or can serve as a bridge to arousal and intercourse.

than a pro forma peck, a foot massage that creates nice sensations on Tina's tired feet, lying on the couch cuddling with intertwined legs, holding hands when going for a walk, taking a moment to sensuously caress the partner's face or arm, being easy and playful in touch, especially spontaneous touch.

Tina and Howard have their special scenario. Howard typically wakes very early on Saturday morning. He enjoys doing chores like feeding the animals, doing woodworking, and/or engaging in a light exercise routine. When Tina wakes she opens the door, which is a signal for Howard to put on the coffee. After a wake-up cup, they take a shower and towel each other dry. Tina checks that the children are still asleep and Howard makes sure the phones are turned off. They lock the bedroom door to guard against unexpected interruptions.

Throughout the morning there have been light, teasing touches and jokes mixed with special looks. Tina enjoys Saturday morning sensual touching standing up rather than lying in bed. She especially enjoys kissing, caressing, and playful genital touching in front of the bureau mirror. The visual feedback of seeing themselves reflected in the mirror is a special excitement. For Tina one of the most sensuous elements is touching while semi-clothed rather than nude—she'll put on one of Howard's shirts and partially button it. Genital and nongenital pleasuring is intermixed. About 65-70 percent of their Saturday mornings include intercourse. They like the concept that intercourse is a "special pleasuring technique" which may or may not be included in the experience. Perhaps 10 percent of the time they engage in manual, oral, or rubbing stimulation to orgasm as an alternative way to express sexual pleasure. Other times are sensuous, relaxing, and comfortable and don't proceed to arousal or orgasm. Part of what makes this a special time for Tina and Howard is the unpredictability and variability. It's their special way to make the transition to the weekend, which, after Saturday mornings, is filled with social and family activities. This is a pattern they developed when their children were school age and continues now when they have visiting grandchildren.

NONDEMAND PLEASURING DURING STRESSFUL TIMES

All couples go through stressful and taxing periods. External circumstances could include a major work deadline, the illness or death of a parent, illness or crisis involving a child, moving or home remodeling, a financial crisis, a period of depression or anxiety. There are times when one or both partners simply do not feel sexual. Sexuality is not a biological need like food or drink. You can cease being sexual for a period of time and nothing untoward will happen to your body. What can and does happen is a strain on the marital bond. One of the best ways to maintain an intimate physical connection during periods of nonsexuality, whether it extends over days, weeks, or months, is to engage in nondemand pleasuring.

Karen and Pete. Karen was being treated for back strain. During the treatment a medication was improperly administered and she was temporarily paralyzed. This was a very frightening experience, and it took seven months before she was fully ambulatory. During this period, Karen was devoid of sexual feelings—she viewed her body with great concern and felt that it had betrayed her. However, her needs for affection, especially her need to be held, was quite high. Pete was used to thinking of touching in primarily sexual terms, so this forced experience of nonsexual, affectionate touching was new to him. Emotionally and physically Pete tried to support Karen. Although they hope never to have to go through a period like that again, they came through it a closer couple. The experience opened Pete to the importance of touch as a means of communicating affection and support.

Sexual dysfunction certainly strains a marital bond. However, couples who maintain affectionate and sensual connection find that this helps to sustain motivation and emotional closeness. Couples who shut off all forms of physical communication are more vulnerable to feelings of isolation and alienation, and are less motivated to deal with marital and sexual problems. In his clinical work, Barry is always encouraged when he sees couples who maintain a touching relationship no matter how severe the sexual dysfunction. These couples have a better prognosis.

MALE-FEMALE DIFFERENCES IN NONDEMAND PLEASURING

It cannot be emphasized enough how the male-female pre-marital double standard interferes with communication between a husband and wife. In traditional male socialization, touch is sexual and always goal-oriented. Women traditionally have valued affectionate touch, but vetoed sexual activity. These rigid roles and definitions are antithetical to our view that nondemand pleasuring can be initiated by either partner. There is no place for hidden agendas, manipulation, teasing, or coercion. Nondemand pleasuring requires a comfort with communicating, verbally and nonverbally, your feelings and desires. The spouse feels free to communicate her feelings and wants. You trust that your partner will respect your feelings. Men can learn to value affectionate and sensual touch for itself, and women can learn to be comfortable with sexual initiation and transition into genital arousal and intercourse. Conversely, a man needs to learn to be comfortable saying no if he does not want to proceed to intercourse. He can say no without feeling he's failed as a male. A woman can let go and be aware of the range of her sensual and sexual feelings rather than being afraid her spouse will push her and that she has to monitor his arousal. Ideally in a marital relationship both people can initiate, suggest alternatives, be open to feelings, and enjoy affection, sensuality, and sexual expression. The nondemand pleasuring concept works best in the context of an emotionally intimate and secure relationship. Nondemand touching has a reciprocal connection, both stimulating and reinforcing intimacy.

CLOSING THOUGHTS

Nondemand pleasuring builds and reinforces comfort with touch, sexual desire, receptivity to sexual stimulation, and emotional intimacy. It can serve as a bridge to sexual arousal, intercourse, and orgasm. Nondemand pleasuring is a solid foundation for intimacy and sexuality in marriage. However, the traditional male objection is correct: nondemand pleasuring is not enough. What men, and women, need to be aware of is that nondemand pleasuring is necessary, but not sufficient, for sexual satisfaction. The next chapter on eroticizing marriage will discuss multiple stimulation scenarios that are necessary, but without the base of nondemand pleasuring, may be difficult to integrate into marital sex.

4
EROTICIZING MARRIAGE

People seldom associate the term "erotic" with marriage. Erotic is associated with new, intense relationships, whether premarital or extramarital. Erotica connotes the "fun, but dirty" sex found in X-rated movies, sex magazines, sex shops, and kinky sex. Can marital sex be erotic? Is this an unrealistic expectation and performance demand? We are absolutely convinced—theoretically, empirically, and in terms of our own marriage—that sex in marriage can be exciting, erotic, and satisfying. We have been married twenty-three years and the quality of our sexual expression is higher than in our early years. Marital sex not only can be erotic, but eroticism is vital if you want to maintain pleasure, playfulness, and sexual satisfaction in your marriage.

In our ideal model of marital sex there would be an emotionally intimate and secure bond that had a solid foundation in nondemand pleasuring. Multiple stimulation is the additional ingredient that serves to eroticize marriage. Multiple stimulation involves giving and/or receiving more than one type of sexual stimulation. In the "traditional" sexual scenario—although we don't believe many couples actually practiced this—the man stimulated the woman until she sufficiently lubricated, then he initiated intercourse and thrusted until they had a simultaneous orgasm (viewed as "ideal sex"). Our guess is that the "traditional" scenario worked for less than 10 percent of couples.

Each couple develops their own style of sexual expression. There is no one right way to eroticize marriage. We will discuss guidelines used by couples who report a high degree of sexual satisfaction and describe exercises developed in the context of sex therapy so that you have a *smorgasbord* of alternatives to talk about and experiment with. The focus is to help you choose sexual scenarios and techniques that add an erotic component to your marital bond.

It is not technique alone, or even primarily, that serves to eroticize marital sex. Marital sex is enhanced by a sense of spontaneity, playfulness, and experimentation, but above all an awareness of your feelings and an openness to creative expression. Sexual creativity emanates from three sources: an awareness of personal feelings and sexual thoughts, a dynamic view of the relationship which includes touching and nonverbal cues, and an openness to experimenting with sexual techniques and scenarios. Creative sex means being aware of your feelings and desires at the time. Take the risk to convey these to your spouse and play them out. You don't need to give a Hollywood-level performance, but you do need to be open to sharing feelings and sexual expression.

The death knell for sexuality is routine and alienation. The most typical sexual scenario for married couples is sex at eleven or later at night. One person, usually the male, reaches over to kiss or caress and says, "Are you up for it?" The sexual interaction follows a standard routine of five to ten minutes of foreplay, during which he tries to get her ready for intercourse; two to eight minutes of intercourse until the man and sometimes the woman reaches orgasm; a minute or two of hugging and talking, and then sleep. Is there something inherently wrong with that scenario? Certainly not. However, it is not the stuff of an erotic and satisfying sexual relationship. Why should sex be the last thing at night after you've finished all the important tasks of life like paying bills, cleaning the house, putting children to sleep, and watching the evening news? When sex becomes the lowest priority in your life, it's hard for it to remain

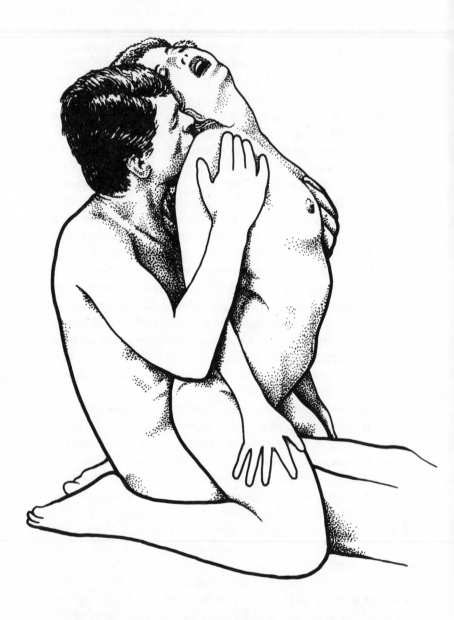

You can enjoy a range of sexual scenarios, positions and pleasuring techniques. Be open to trying different positions and types of pleasuring.

satisfying, much less erotic. A necessary component for erotic sex is setting aside time to be sexual. The couple needs to be alert and awake, to value the time and privacy, and to anticipate coming together for intimate sexual expression.

Some people are offended by the concept of a "couple date." They feel sex should be totally spontaneous. Spontaneity is to be valued, but in a couple's busy life, between children, jobs, household chores, community responsibilities, friends, and extended family, if you don't set aside couple time it won't happen. Couple time doesn't mean having sex each time you are together, but it does mean setting aside time to be together without distractions. This special time allows the interaction to be sexual, but is not a sexual demand. Spontaneity works better in movies and novels than in a busy couple's life. It is easier to be spontaneous on vacations or weekends than at home during the busy week.

An interesting side note is that extramarital affairs have an air of excitement, anticipation, and eroticism. Yet engaging in an affair requires an enormous amount of planning and arrangement. You need to decide where to meet—often at a hotel or motel—and be assertive enough to ask for the "day rate." You block off time in your schedule, cover yourself at work, have someone pick up children, and plan what to tell your spouse if she calls. Not exactly a spontaneous coming together. Spontaneity can be fun and erotic, but its role is overemphasized. Spontaneous sexuality doesn't appear out of nowhere—there is a sense of connection and being together that allows a low-key tone to change into a passionate, erotic, sexual coming together.

A crucial concept in creative sexuality is that quality is more important than quantity. Couples—as in the Woody Allen movie *Annie Hall*—consistently argue over frequency of intercourse. These discussions are counterproductive and self-defeating. Sexual satisfaction is not measured by frequency or by the number of orgasms. The best measure of sexual satisfaction is a sense of giving and receiving pleasure and feeling intimately bonded. This comes from quality, not quantity. One element of erotic feeling is recalling special sexual experiences with the spouse.

What makes for good sexual quality? An important component is the development and refinement of sexual scenarios. Each individual and couple will have their favorite sexual scenario(s). Some people find the best time to be sexual is when they wake up. Others prefer sex after coffee and the morning paper. Others like a "nooner," before or after a nap, before dinner (sex as an appetizer) or after dinner (sex as dessert). Part of the sexual scenario is setting a conducive sensual mood. Couples set that mood by listening to music, going for a walk, talking about pleasant moments, having a glass of wine by candlelight, taking a bath together, having fifteen minutes of alone time and then getting together, or by her meeting him at the door in a sexy outfit with an invitation to come into the bedroom. Other couples prefer doing something together like working in the garden, talking about feelings, or working out and then making the transition to being sexual. Many creative couples prefer to start the scenario outside the bedroom. They begin sensual touching and play in the living room or den and don't move into the bedroom until both are feeling sexual.

Once the scenario is initiated, couples prefer different ways to play it out. Remember, there's no question of right or wrong, you have only to act on your feelings and desires. Sometimes people enjoy taking turns, with one as the primary giver of pleasure, while other couples prefer mutual stimulation. Some people verbally express feelings and make requests. Others would rather let their fingers do the talking. Many couples prefer the scenario of moving from slow, tender, nongenital touching, to light, playful, genital stimulation, and then to more focused, erotic, multiple stimulation, before proceeding to intercourse. Other couples begin intercourse as early as possible in the scenario. Most couples prefer multiple stimulation, both during the pleasuring period and intercourse itself. Other couples find it more erotic if they focus on one form of stimulation at a time and receive the maximum pleasure from that. For some, manual stimulation is most arousing, for some oral stimulation, and for others rubbing. Some couples prefer using one or two intercourse positions, others enjoy using a variety and changing positions during intercourse. Creative sex means being aware of your feelings and preferences. Develop and play out sexual scenarios that are erotic for you. Quality depends on keeping open channels of sexual communication, whether by verbal requests, nonverbal hand-guiding, moving your body, or guiding your partner's mouth, hand, or body.

ORAL-GENITAL SEX

The major revolution in sexual technique has been in experimentation with oral-genital sex. About 75 percent of married couples will try oral sex and for approximately 40 percent oral sex is a regular part of their sexual repertoire. This makes perfect sense—the mouth and genitals are the two parts of the body most capable of giving and receiving sexual pleasure. Couples who engage in oral sex report heightened sexual satisfaction, including greater enjoyment of intercourse.

Why does oral sex have a reputation as "kinky" or "dirty?" Much of the problem comes from our use, and misuse, of sexual language. The formal terms "cunnilingus" (the man kissing, licking, or sucking the woman's vulva) and "fellatio" (her kissing, licking, or sucking his penis) are such cold, awkward Latin words. Slang phrases such as "blow job," "go down on," "suck off," "eat me," and "69" have hostile and/ or derogatory connotations. Oral sex has traditionally been viewed as "exciting, but dirty." Is it something you would do with an intimate partner? When married men go to prostitutes they are more likely to request fellatio than intercourse. Are their wives too inhibited to give oral sex, are men too embarrassed to ask, or do they believe only a prostitute could do it right? Some believe that only men who are insecure about their penises would perform cunnilingus. They fear that a woman might become hooked on oral sex and forgo intercourse. Or that the woman who has orgasms through cunnilingus can't have an orgasm during intercourse. What a lot of nonsense. Couples can develop comfort with oral sex scenarios and experiment with oral sex techniques which add a creative and erotic component to their sexual life.

In experimenting with oral-genital sexuality, as with any sexual technique, a crucial guideline is to be open to experimentation, but not to allow coercion. The focus is on pleasure, not performance. You don't need to prove anything to anybody. The best way to approach oral stimulation is gradually, intermixing it with manual stimulation. We suggest bathing or showering together first to avoid worry about being unclean or genital smells. Couples who don't have time or who don't want to bother with a shower can use a washcloth and deodorant soap to clean their genitals.

We suggest beginning with a giver-receiver format. The receiver can close his or her eyes, which reduces self-consciousness as well as helps you focus on pleasurable sensations. Begin oral stimulation with kissing before moving to licking and sucking. He can lightly kiss and run his tongue around the vulva, exploring the labia before focusing on the clitoral area. The woman might kiss and run her tongue along the shaft of his penis before kissing or sucking on the glans. The giver can feel free to experiment with a range of oral stimulation techniques. If there is discomfort or pain, the recipient needs to say that so the partner can change the type of stimulation. The recipient can enjoy the sensations and take in the pleasure.

Once you've established a basic comfort with giving and receiving oral stimulation, experiment with scenarios and positions to build erotic sensations. Some people enjoy passively receiving, but the majority find it more arousing to move their body in a rhythmic manner while being stimulated. Changing positions can increase erotic feelings. Many women prefer the man to kneel beside her rather than lie between her legs, so that she can touch him and feel more connected. Many men prefer the position of man standing, woman kneeling, because it gives him freedom to move and touch her as she's stimulating him. Some couples enjoy mutual oral-genital stimulation (the "69" position) as the ultimate in multiple stimulation while others find it distracting to give and receive at the same time. There is no right or wrong position or technique. State your preferences, be aware of your partner's comfort, and play around until you develop a quality oral sex scenario(s).

A common fear among women is losing control or gagging during fellatio. To prevent gagging we suggest two techniques.

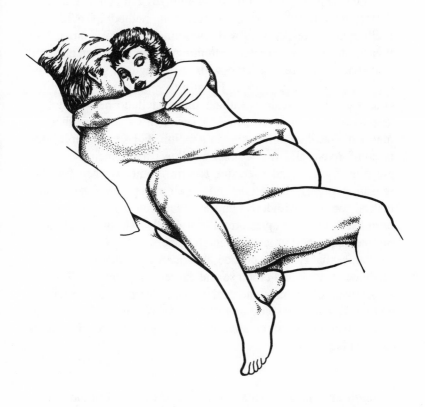

Side-by-side intercourse allows for greater touching and communications. Multiple stimulation during intercourse increases erotic sensations.

Guide the penis to the side of your mouth, toward your cheek, rather than putting it down the center. The second is to keep your hand on the penis so insertion is not too deep or fast. Holding his penis gives you a sense of control during fellatio as well as providing him additional stimulation.

Is oral sex strictly a pleasuring technique or can it proceed to orgasm? Being orgasmic during cunnilingus can facilitate arousal during intercourse. The most common method of achieving multiorgasmic response is with cunnilingus. Many women find it easier to be orgasmic with cunnilingus than intercourse. Some find that if they're orgasmic with cunnilingus it's easier to be orgasmic during intercourse. Fellatio to orgasm is a more difficult issue. If the male ejaculates during fellatio he will not be able to continue to intercourse. A sensitive issue is whether the man will ejaculate in the woman's mouth. For some couples this is comfortable and the woman swallows the semen (semen is hygienically safe and even low caloric). Other women find the sensation of semen gushing into their mouth unpleasant, and instead the man withdraws and ejaculates on the sheet, on her, or himself. Other couples prefer to use fellatio only as a pleasuring technique and proceed to intercourse.

Oral sexuality can enhance the quality of marital sex and facilitate creative and erotic sexual expression. The couple needs to be aware of feelings and desires, communicate these verbally and nonverbally, develop oral sex scenarios that are comfortable and arousing, and be creative in integrating oral sex into their lovemaking.

Sandi and Jack. Couples who find sex easy from the beginning need to be aware of the potential trap of taking it for granted and allowing the sexual relationship to stagnate. Sandi met Jack when she was twenty-three and he twenty-four. Their prior dating and sexual experiences followed the typical roller-coaster pattern of excitement and anticipation at the beginning, highs and lows throughout, and pain and hurt at the breakup. Both felt lucky that they'd avoided destructive people and used effective contraception. When they met at a wedding, both were ready for a more serious relationship. Although they still disagree about who pursued whom, the first two months were romantic and erotic. Romantic love is a special experience not to be missed, although it is not a good basis for a mature marital choice. This is a passionate and fun time, full of special moments and idealization of the person and relationship. Sandi and Jack did special things lovers do—called at three in the morning, made love in the woods on a camping trip, stayed up all night sharing their hopes and dreams, had sex three times a day, and swore they'd never hurt or disappoint the other. Romantic love is an exhilarating experience, but it's based on a fantasy view of the partner, love, and sex. Romantic love seldom lasts even for a year. Sandi looks back on those months more wistfully than Jack, although he too has fond memories.

After the romantic love phase turned into the more mature, stable, and lasting state of intimacy, sexuality remained easy and high quality. Both experienced sexual desire, although Jack's was more easily elicited. Both were easily aroused, were receptive and responsive to stimulation, and one's arousal increased the other's. Orgasm was readily achieved, although on occasion Jack would ejaculate earlier than desired, and in those cases would manually stimulate Sandi. After sex they felt warm and bonded. Their marriage was a true celebration with family and friends very supportive. Getting pregnant was not a problem; they had a girl and boy without any difficulties and then Jack had a vasectomy. Their life sailed along and they were viewed as a "golden couple."

One of the realities of life is that hard times come to all couples. You cannot avoid difficulties, and it's no use pretending that they're not happening. Accept the reality of the situation, cope with it, and engage in problem-solving as a couple. In an eight-month period Sandi's mother died, their son broke his arm, Jack's business was in a trough and he had to take a significant pay cut, and Sandi had a short affair with a doctor she'd met at the hospital. The affair came to light when Jack discovered her diaphragm and confronted her about its use since he'd had a vasectomy. The marital bond of respect, trust, and intimacy had been damaged in many ways. An extramarital

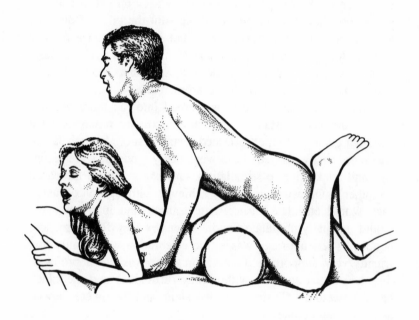

You can use pillows or cushions to increase comfort and sensations during rear-entry intercourse. Don't be afraid to experiment with your intimate partner.

affair shakes the bond and plunges the marriage into crisis. The wife's having an affair is a reversal of the male-female double standard and the husband reacts as if it's an attack on his masculinity and sexual adequacy. Jack was hurt and angry, and because of his career and financial setbacks as well, felt extremely insecure and vulnerable. Sandi herself had felt vulnerable at the time and the affair had been an impulsive one. She regretted it and was apologetic, and was particularly distressed by Jack's feelings of betrayal and the damage to their marital trust. The better the marriage, the more negative is the impact of an affair.

Sandi and Jack found the next three months the hardest of their marriage. In addition to dealing with the other issues in their lives, they had to work through feelings of betrayal, anger, and depression, and rebuild the trust bond. Sex during those three months was particularly difficult. Like most married couples, Sandi and Jack had treated their sexual relationship with benign neglect. Sex is like a garden, it needs consistent attention and care. It was not that sex was dysfunctional, but that it had settled into a routine: less frequent, late at night, with less feeling and involvement and fewer special experiences. Sex following the revelation of the affair was sometimes angry, as if Jack was trying to get back at Sandi and hard, rapid thrusting was his weapon. Other times when they tried to be sexual there was a tentativeness that made them feel as if they were "walking on eggshells." The automatic, easy sex was gone.

Although a crisis hastens the demise of easy unself-conscious sexual expression, the truth is that it eventually disappears from all, even the best marriages. Sandi and Jack were abruptly confronted with a transition all couples need to face—how to integrate creative, quality sex into their ongoing marriage. Rather than trying to return to the "good old days," they were better off focusing their energy on developing a couple sexual style that, in the long run, would be of higher quality.

For Sandi and Jack, as with other couples in crisis, seeking marital therapy was the best thing they could do for themselves. It helped them to deal with the affair as well as other marital issues, and mobilized them to get on with the task of revitalizing their bond. The therapist's first suggestion was to put a temporary prohibition on intercourse and other orgasm-oriented activity and encourage nongenital pleasuring. Sandi found that Jack's touching her in a nonhostile, tender, nondemanding manner greatly increased her sense of attraction and desire to be with him. At first, Jack had difficulty being open to Sandi's touch, but as he did his resentment and desperateness began to disappear. Nondemand touching and sensuality were the foundations for their renewed sexual bond.

Genital stimulation was reintroduced a week before the therapist lifted the ban on intercourse. This allowed Sandi and Jack to experiment with genital stimulation to orgasm, something they had not done since their premarital years. Nondemand pleasuring builds comfort and sensuality. Varied and creative genital stimulation adds a sense of eroticism and adventure to sexual expression. The genuine enjoyment of genital stimulation scenarios made for a very sexual week. Even without intercourse, or maybe because there was a ban on intercourse, their sexual expression was more creative and erotic than it had been for years. Jack discovered a pleasuring position in which he knelt on the bed facing Sandi, who was also kneeling. This allowed him to engage in oral breast stimulation combined with manual clitoral stimulation while she stimulated his penis. For the first time in their marriage, Sandi was multiorgasmic. Although Jack was embarrassed about ejaculating in her hand, the sensations of direct stimulation to orgasm were exciting and gratifying.

When the therapist lifted the ban on intercourse she strongly suggested that Sandi and Jack rethink the role of intercourse, viewing intercourse as a special pleasuring technique. The pleasuring positions, techniques, and scenarios could be continued and integrated with intercourse. Eroticizing marriage means incorporating multiple stimulation throughout lovemaking, before and during intercourse. She warned them not to revert to the standard "foreplay" routine they'd grown accustomed to, but to continue with creative pleasuring scenarios, positions, and stimulation techniques. Intercourse was a natural extension of the pleasuring process.

The second focus was on continuing multiple stimulation during intercourse. Sandi particularly desired manual clitoral stimulation in combination with intercourse. As well, she enjoyed kissing during coital thrusting, and having her breasts caressed. Jack enjoyed doing this and focusing on visual stimulation. He found it arousing to look at Sandi as she became more excited. Jack also enjoyed closing his eyes and focusing on sexual fantasies. Marital sex benefits from multiple stimulation and eroticism during intercourse.

TAKING RISKS WITH YOUR SPOUSE

Sexual thoughts, fantasies, and feelings are some of the most private and sensitive aspects of human existence. An advantage of an intimate relationship is sharing these. People fear rejection, or fear that their requests will be perceived as "kinky" or even perverse. We encourage couples to be open in stating their sexual feelings and requests. A key to sexual intimacy is trusting your partner and being able to make clear and direct sexual requests. He needs to hear it as a request, not a demand. This gives the spouse freedom to say, "Let's try it," to offer an alternative stimulation technique, or to say, "No, I'm not comfortable with it." For example, a woman had read about being stimulated by a feather and was interested in trying it, but her husband disliked the lightweight of feathers. He suggested instead rubbing a string of pearls over her body. A man wanted his hands and feet tied with heavy rope, but his spouse suggested instead knots made with yarn. Don't do something which is coercive, causes pain, or is not personally comfortable. Within those guidelines there are a number of scenarios, positions, and techniques that can be explored and experimented with. Taking sexual risks will pay dividends in higher quality, more erotic marital sexual expression.

Jill and Ron. This was a couple who tried to "keep up with the Joneses," whether in buying new video equipment, seeing the most avant-garde play, reading trendy novels, or trying the newest gourmet cuisine. Each year, as soon as they read or heard about a new sexual scenario to experiment with, they would try it. In the days before AIDS it was anal intercourse, then it was use of fruit-flavored creams with oral sex, then came X-rated videos to use during lovemaking, followed by X-rated motels with special movies, Jacuzzis, vibrating beds, mirrors, and last year it was playing out sexual fantasies with all the accouterments, including clothing and music. Still, Jill and Ron felt that their sex life was stale, and were on the lookout for the next sexually sophisticated scenario.

In talking with a friend who was a traditional marital therapist, they were confronted with the fact that these techniques did not make their sex life more erotic. He told them they were substituting external stimulation for an exploration of their internal feelings and what they really wanted from each other. The next day Jill suggested taking a walk and talking about this observation. Ron, on the defensive, said that their friend was old-fashioned. Jill agreed, but the more she thought about it the more she realized that she wasn't doing what she felt like sexually. They would try something for a while, but then drop it. Why was that? As Ron thought about it, he realized that what he liked best was having his testicles rubbed while Jill orally stimulated him. Yet she hadn't done that in over a year and he hadn't asked her to. Jill said the scenario she liked best was pretty basic: lying on her back with Ron kneeling over her rubbing his penis against her breast while manually stimulating her clitoral area. She felt embarrassed at desiring something so "normal," so she didn't request it. It was hard for Jill and Ron to accept that the essence of creative, erotic sexuality is found by focusing on feelings and preferences, not learning some exotic or sophisticated technique. Jill said it best: "We were so involved in trying to prove we were sexually liberated that we stopped communicating our intimate sexual needs."

CLOSING THOUGHTS

The key to eroticizing marriage is an awareness of your unique couple sexual style and being able to communicate sexual feelings and requests. We encourage an open attitude of experimentation with different sexual scenarios, positions, and stimulation techniques, especially multiple stimulation during intercourse. Creative, high-quality sexuality is much more than technique. Be aware of your feelings and erotic preferences and communicate these. The combination of emotional intimacy, nondemand pleasuring, and multiple stimulation is the best way to maintain erotic and satisfying marital sex.

5
EQUALITY BETWEEN THE SEXES

Among single people the "Dating Game" is more like the "War Between the Sexes." A tragedy for American couples is that the self-defeating attitudes, behavior, and emotional reactions learned premaritally serve to sabotage their marriage.

What is needed is a new awareness of female-male relationships to facilitate respect, trust, and intimacy. The traditional double standard held that men and women were different, especially sexually, and needed to assume separate and rigid roles in marriage. We are unequivocally opposed to the double standard. It fosters a climate of disrespect and miscommunication. Its only advantage is that the rules about male-female roles although wrong—are simple and clear. The radical feminist standard of absolute equality between women and men, with everything split fifty-fifty, sets unrealistic expectations and results in constant power struggles. The male is viewed as the "bad guy." Traditional men call those who cave in to feminist demands "wimps." The radical feminist approach downplays trust and intimacy and overemphasizes personal independence and the distribution of power. This makes for better political polemics than a model for a secure and intimate marriage. What is needed is a new model that conceptualizes female-male relationships in a manner that will enhance psychological and sexual well-being for both sexes and provides a basis for a respectful, trusting, and intimate marriage.

A MODEL OF EQUITY BETWEEN WOMEN AND MEN

The foundation of this model is that each brings to the relationship the self-concept of a person deserving respect, and being trustworthy, autonomous, competent, and sexual. You cannot expect your partner to give this to you. You need to assume personal responsibility for developing positive self-esteem, including sexual self-esteem. Well-functioning marriages are based on a positive influence model. The marriage serves to bring out the best in you as a person.

The model is not one of equality in every aspect of life, which is overly idealistic and doomed to failure. A more solid, realistic, and satisfying base is a sense of equity in the marital relationship. One person can have prime responsibility and skill in a specific area while the other has prime responsibility and skill in a different area. The crucial element is that the couple relate as respectful human beings who value each other's competence and share power in an equitable manner. When the couple relate as respectful, trusting, and caring people, they offer an excellent model from which children can learn about female-male relationships and marriage. An added bonus is that people who treat each other well outside the bedroom will usually treat each other well inside the bedroom.

Respect is the cornerstone of the equity model. You need to respect yourself and the way you are in the relationship as well as respecting your partner. When respect begins to erode, the marital bond is in danger. Respect is based on genuine knowledge of yourself and your spouse; you are accepted for your weaknesses as well as your strengths.

A second crucial dimension involves trust. Instead of there being a war between the sexes with each jealously guarding his or her turf, in a trusting relationship you have confidence that the spouse would not do something to purposely undercut or harm you. You view him as having your best interests at heart and as your friend and supporter. This does not mean returning to the traditional traps of a woman naïvely accepting everything a man does and him putting her on a pedestal. Discuss and make an explicit agreement about what you mean by the trust bond and how important that bond is in your marriage. Too many wives have felt victimized by husbands they naïvely believed and who took advantage of them. Too many husbands have felt devastated and abandoned by wives who they believed would love and stand by them no matter what.

This process needs to begin before marriage. Choose a spouse who is deserving of trust. Have a clear understanding about the importance of trust in the marital bond. Trust is not something you can or should take for granted, it needs to be firmly established and its importance reinforced. For trust to be genuine, it must be reciprocal.

Even though there is a trust bond, at times there will be problems, disappointments, and anger in dealing with issues and disagreements. That is the reality of the complex process of marriage. In dealing with mundane as well as major issues, each person needs to communicate clearly, discuss feelings and perceptions, suggest alternatives, and problem solve so that agreements are reached that both can live with. In dealing with difficult issues, it is important that you trust your partner's intentions. Refrain from doing something that hurts intentionally.

Discussions can break down into power struggles in which you care more about the fight than preserving the fabric of the relationship. When power struggles degenerate, they become "pissing contests," and the issue is no longer important. In fact, you forget the original, and the issue becomes not to lose. Power struggles are destructive to the trust bond. Couples can deal with difficult issues and reach agreements in ways that reinforce rather than damage this bond. You can state your feelings, perceptions, and requests in a clear and forceful manner without breaking trust. Negotiating and problem solving does not break trust as long as you are acting in your best interests and are not trying to intimidate or coerce your partner. Do not negotiate to win the battle but lose the war, but to reach an agreement. Ideally, you should feel good about the process and outcome, and, minimally, you should be able to live with the agreement without feeling undercut by your spouse.

Trust means more than not having an extramarital affair. Sexual fidelity is not the only, or even the most important, element in marital trust. Extramarital affairs are a highly emotional and value-laden topic, and we have devoted an entire chapter to this issue. Our suggestion is to develop a prior agreement regarding trust and the issue of extramarital affairs.

The third important aspect of equity is emotional and sexual intimacy. Traditional, as well as modern, mythology holds that men and women are very different creatures when it comes to emotional and sexual expression. Women are purported to be more sensitive, empathic, able to express sadness, and dependent on being in a loving relationship in order to have sexual feelings. Men are purported to value control and rationality, are able to express only anger, and value sexuality more highly than anything else in marriage. Women are said to value love and allow sex, and men to value sex and allow marriage to obtain sex. What rubbish!

The model of emotional and sexual intimacy we propose emphasizes that for a well-functioning couple each partner needs to be comfortable and expressive both ways. Each can self-disclose, express a range of feelings, share perceptions, problem solve, reach agreements, and be emotionally vulnerable and open. Emotional caring should be deep and stable as well as loving and intense. Emotional attraction includes a belief that you can live a shared life.

Sexuality is integral to intimacy. Intimacy includes sexual expression as well as sharing thoughts, feelings, beliefs, values, and plans. Sexuality is a positive, integral component of marriage. Sex serves to reinforce and deepen intimacy, is a shared pleasure, and serves as a tension reducer or safety valve, but contrary to the media myth, it is not the most important element in a marriage. When sex goes well, it's no more than 15-20 percent of the marriage, with its most important function being to energize the marital bond. It is only when sex is dysfunctional or part of a power struggle that it plays the inordinately powerful role of robbing the relationship of intimacy and draining away loving feelings.

Sexuality works best in a marriage where there is a sense of emotional and sexual equity. Each partner can feel comfortable initiating (this is particularly hard for women) and each can feel free to say no (this is particularly hard for men). Sex is more than genitals, intercourse, and the few seconds of orgasm. Sexuality involves acceptance of yourself as a sexual person, comfort with nondemand touching inside and outside the bedroom, enjoyment of sensuality, responsivity to genital stimulation, openness to multiple stimulation, the ability to let go and be orgasmic, and emotional satisfaction. Sex serves as an important expression of intimacy and as a bonding experience. It has been said that "a marriage can tolerate bad sex, but it's hard to survive no sex." The couple need to view each other as sexual people with sexuality integrated into a respectful, trusting, and intimate marriage.

The most intimate and stable relationship between a woman and a man is marriage. Although elements of the equity model are relevant to a range of interactions between women and men, including work relationships, friendships, parenting, and other social and family relationships, it is most crucial in marriage. These are our guidelines for equity between the sexes:

1. Base relationships between women and men on respectful attitudes that promote, and even demand, equity.
2. Maintain open and flexible attitudes toward female-male roles.
3. Work toward an acceptance and security about yourself and your femininity or masculinity so that you do not need the approval of the opposite sex nor are you intimidated by others.
4. Be aware that intellectually, behaviorally, emotionally, and sexually there are more similarities than differences between women and men.
5. Encourage personal and/or professional friendships with the opposite sex, but resist the pressure to sexualize these relationships.

6. Be comfortable and confident in your femininity or masculinity so that activities or interests which have been labeled as belonging to the opposite sex can be integrated into your life.

7. Understand that an intimate sexual relationship will be more satisfying if both the woman and man can initiate, say no, request, and enjoy a range of sexual pleasures.

8. Acknowledge that conception, contraception, and children are as much the responsibility of men as women.

9. Cultivate a marriage based on respect, equity, trust, and intimacy for the most satisfaction for both women and men.

10. Promote a communicative, sharing, and giving relationship for emotional and sexual satisfaction.

Couples who live out these guidelines, sharing responsibility to implement them, can avoid the ongoing war between the sexes and enjoy a satisfying and stable marriage.

DIFFERENCES BETWEEN WOMEN AND MEN

Much of the discussion and writing concerning female-male roles has been ideological, moralistic, and highly emotional. It generates much heat but little light. Let us approach this most complex subject from a more objective, scientific viewpoint. There has been a great deal of scientific research during the past twenty years about female-male similarities and differences along a number of dimensions—physical strength, intellectual functioning, behavioral characteristics, health, sexual response, emotional reactivity, and interpersonal traits. The objective evidence is overwhelming: there are many more similarities than differences between women and men in all dimensions, including sexual response. The same phases of desire, arousal, orgasm, and emotional satisfaction are experienced by both women and men. The same psychological process of positive anticipation, the same physiological process of arousal via vasocongestion and myotonia (muscle spasm), the same rhythmic contractions of orgasm, and the same gradual resolution period occurs for women and men. Of course there are differences, but the similarities—physically, psychologically, and emotionally —vastly outnumber them.

The sexual differences involve latency of response and variability of orgasm. Women require a longer period of time and more direct genital stimulation for arousal than men, although these differences decrease with age and experience. Female orgasmic response is more flexible and variable. The male has a single orgasm which is accompanied by ejaculation. The woman might be nonorgasmic, singly orgasmic, or multiorgasmic. This might occur in the pleasuring/foreplay period, during intercourse, or in the afterplay phase. This does not mean female sexual response is better or worse than male, only that it is more complex and variable. The important similarity is that both women and men are sexual people with the ability to give and receive pleasure, to be orgasmic, and to perceive sexuality as a positive part of life and an enhancement of an intimate relationship.

Marlene and Paul. Few couples have benefited from growing up in families where there was a positive equitable model between mother and father. Marlene and Paul were in the large majority who desired to develop their marital bond in a very different manner from that of their parents.

Marlene was ten when her parents separated. She observed the three-year agony of their trying to reconcile, angrily parting, and trying again. Her father left for the final time when she was thirteen, after a violent confrontation in which her mother called the police—which she had done previously, but this time followed through with legal charges. Marlene had minimal contact with her father until she was twenty-two. He had remarried and his life was more stable, although he would still lose his temper and lash out at his new wife and child. Marlene saw her father as a successful professional person, but as a man who was dependent on a woman to keep his life on track. She resented his temper and was frightened by it. She feared men would use physical intimidation and anger to get their way with her, too. She was more empathic with her mother, although as an adolescent she used her mother's emotional weakness as leverage to get her way. Looking back, Marlene was not proud of her adolescent behavior.

Like many other children of divorce, Marlene had a strong need to marry and develop a more stable situation than she had grown up with. Negative motivation seldom, if ever, promotes positive behavior. Marlene's marriage at age twenty-one was a badly thought-out choice. One of the reasons children of divorce have higher divorce rates themselves is that they marry young and idealize their partner as the perfect romantic love object. Marriage needs to be viewed as a rational and emotional commitment to sharing a life together. Romantic love subverts making a mature and healthy choice.

Eight months into the marriage, Marlene was badly disillusioned and scared. She had admired her mother's seeking therapy after her divorce, and felt that individual and group therapy had made her mother a stronger person. Marlene entered individual psychotherapy when her husband adamantly refused to seek marital therapy. The therapist was respectful and empathic with Marlene, but confrontative about her taking responsibility for decisions, and evaluating her reasons for marrying and the viability of the marriage. The therapist suggested that Marlene talk to her mother and father for information and consultation, but not to blame them for the state of her life or have them make decisions for her. Each parent was supportive and neither pressed her to stay married.

Being in individual therapy to improve a marriage can be helpful to the individual, but usually increases marital dissatisfaction. Marlene's husband made fun of the therapy and blamed all their marital problems on "immaturity" and "selfishness." Marlene was aware enough to refuse the blame, and was resentful that he wouldn't consider the problems as couple issues. After consulting with friends, family, and her therapist, she decided that rather than allow the relationship to deteriorate further, increasing the pain and allowing things to get more out of control, she had to confront the reality that hers was not a viable marriage. Although this was a sad outcome and there ensued a difficult transition to being single again, Marlene never regretted her decision. She was glad that she lived at a time when women were responsible for themselves and didn't have to cling to a destructive marriage. Marlene did not need a man in her life in order to feel like a complete person.

Marlene met Paul a year and a half after the divorce. In choosing to marry him, she felt she had learned from the past and was ready to make a marital commitment for the right reasons. Paul too came from a bad parental model, although his parents had remained married. He had read about abusive husbands in magazine articles and seen them depicted on television and in the movies, but he had not heard or read about abusive wives and mothers. Yet this was the reality of his family. Although both parents denied it, alcoholism and drug abuse were the central problems. Paul's father functioned at work, but used alcohol to shut off his feelings and to avoid dealing with the destructive marital and family dynamics. Paul saw his father as a nice person, but too weak to confront difficult, if not impossible, issues. Paul was extremely frightened of his mother. About every two weeks she would have an alcoholic rage, often accompanied by violence toward her husband and children. This could result in anything from a broken chair to a broken arm. Neighbors called the police, who left after things calmed down. Paul's psychological scars from this violence were deeper and more lasting than the scar he bore on his arm. He was determined never to get himself into an abusive or destructive relationship with a woman.

As a young adult, Paul attended meetings and read material about adult children of alcoholics. These efforts increased his awareness and decreased the stigma he felt, but he was not impressed with some of the people in the group. He was wary of making commitments, although he enjoyed dating, sexuality, and "light" relationships.

Marlene and Paul met through mutual friends who encouraged them to volunteer for a Special Olympics project. Marlene was attracted to the open and engaging manner Paul displayed with retarded children. Paul found Marlene very attractive. She seemed competent and self-possessed even when everything around her was chaotic. After the day's activities, a group of volunteers went to a bar to socialize and Marlene and Paul joined them. Paul noted that she limited herself to one drink, as did he. He was impressed by how sociable and down to earth she was. Marlene liked Paul, but was not as taken with him.

In a relationship, someone has to take the risk and be the pursuer. In social scripts it is traditionally the man. Paul asked for Marlene's phone number and called the next day. Marlene had a pattern of making informal first dates during daylight hours, so she suggested that they meet for lunch. Although Paul had suggested a movie, he agreed to lunch. First dates are some of the best and worst parts of being single. They can be disappointing and tiresome. Going through the routine of exchanging information about where you live, your work, where you're from, and what you like, can be tedious. On the positive side, there's the sense of anticipation, excitement, adventure, and hope that this could turn into something special.

Both Marlene and Paul approached a serious relationship with a sense of caution. They had fun getting to know each other. They enjoyed touching and affection, but neither was in a rush to sexualize the relationship. Neither trusted romantic love feelings or intense emotional expression. At the very least, Marlene wanted to be sure that Paul would be a good and trusted friend. Paul was particularly wary of Marlene's turning into an explosive, unpredictable, emotional person.

When their children are old enough to ask about their parents' courtship, the story Marlene and Paul will share begins with a Friday night movie that was so bad they left in the middle. It was a pleasant fall night, and they decided to take a walk along the river. They were discussing mental retardation caused by the mother's alcoholism. Before he knew it, Paul was talking about this in a very personal manner and relating it to his family experience. His self-disclosure was not just an emotional outburst; he asked whether Marlene were interested in hearing the story. They walked and talked for over two hours. This established a pattern that was to last throughout their marriage. Paul found it easier to discuss emotional issues while engaged in an activity like walking, raking leaves, or working on a household project. Marlene was an empathic listener, hearing out his story and feelings rather than feeling sorry for him or rushing in to make him feel better. She disclosed one thing about herself that really struck him—that she believed in marriage and wanted children, but was a complete person as she was. Paul appreciated her strength and was relieved that she did not exhibit the desperateness he saw in so many divorced women. The second part of the walk was quieter, with more kissing and touching. They desired to make love, which Marlene acknowledged. However, she did not want to add a sexual dimension to this already full night. She invited him to spend the night Saturday, after they'd had a day to think things out, and only if Paul were open to a serious relationship.

This would not make a great romantic novel, but it does make a great start for an intimate relationship. Paul brought a change of clothes as well as condoms. Marlene preferred to used a diaphragm, but not until after they had a frank conversation about any possible risk of sexually transmitted disease. She suggested they have sex before dinner. She wasn't looking for a great sexual performance, but an exploration and an introduction.

Once the sense of newness and illicitness wears off, it takes most couples about six months to develop a sexual style that is satisfying for both partners. Marlene and Paul were lucky in that they brought to the relationship positive sexual attitudes, sexual awareness and comfort, and were receptive and responsive to touch. Sexuality was relatively easy for them, but unlike other couples, they did not take it for granted. Especially after two years of marriage, there is a tendency to allow the sexual relationship to rest on its laurels. Marlene and Paul worked together to enhance sexuality so it would energize their marital bond as well as provide special moments and memories of playfulness and passion. Both felt free to initiate and either could say no and offer an alternative. They engaged in nondemand touching both inside and outside the bedroom. Marlene and Paul enjoyed sensual activities like showering together and using lotion or powder to enhance body caresses. They were open to sexual scenarios in which one person was the giver as well as more mutual and interactive scenarios. They enjoyed multiple stimulation, both before and during intercourse. Not all touching led to intercourse. They used a variety of intercourse posi-tions and had a range of scenarios from "quickies" to slow, prolonged lovemaking. They accepted variability in sexual expression—sometimes sex was satisfying for both, sometimes one enjoyed it more than the other, and when it was mediocre or poor they laughed it off rather than blaming or being worried. They enjoyed a range of afterplay experiences. Equity between the sexes occurs both inside and outside the bedroom.

Their decision to marry did not follow the traditional roman-tic script. Marlene and Paul talked about strengths and potential problem areas as individuals and as a couple. Marlene needed assurance that Paul was committed to making the marriage successful, and Paul needed assurance that Marlene's interest was genuine and would not change with marriage. They would not tolerate the unsatisfying patterns of their parents' marriages—they would not stay married if their relationship degenerated. They used this attitude not as a way out, but as positive motiva-tion to enhance their marital bond and keep it viable. Marriage and sexuality is a process, not a product—it requires continual time, energy, commitment, and openness to change and growth.

The decision to marry needs to be based on both emotional and rational factors. In addition to a sense of intimacy and sexual attraction, you believe you can build a satisfying life together. Marlene and Paul talked about a five-year plan for their lives and marriage: where they would live, how they would handle career and money issues, that they would wait at least two years before having a child, that both would be actively involved in parenting, that each had freedom to pursue individual interests and friends but not to have sexual affairs or to do things that were detrimental to the marriage. They dis-cussed hard issues such as the psychological "traps" from their parents' marriages, Marlene's divorce, Paul's fear of a serious commitment, dealing with in-laws, how to argue and reach agreements, and the difficulties inherent in balancing individual interests, two careers, their marital bond, and parenting chil-dren. Love and intimacy is not enough for a successful mar-riage. Both partners need to be aware and committed to deal with issues, to talk out problems before they lead to emotional alienation or a crisis. Marlene and Paul realized that there are no perfect people or perfect marriages. However, they had a strong commitment to make their marriage an equitable, satisfying, and stable one.

Marlene and Paul have been married eighteen years; Teresa is fifteen and Mike twelve. They emphasize equity in their marriage. Sometimes it has worked "like in the book." The best example is that Paul's career has gone better than either would have predicted. He was in a position to take more risks, since Marlene's job as a bank operations officer provided a steady source of income. Paul had an advanced degree in biomedical engineering and developed and sold instrument patents to a hospital supply company. They respected each other's professional competence, and approached financial matters as a team.

The area in which the equity guidelines worked least well involved house maintenance. Paul did not keep his agreements about cooking and house cleaning. In truth, he was a terrible cook. On his nights to cook they invariably had carry-out food or salads from the grocery store. Marlene was not happy about this, but realized that it was not likely to change. The guidelines worked well around parenting. Paul was a more involved and responsible parent than either had expected. He felt equally comfortable nurturing as providing guidance and discipline. This freed Marlene to expand her role from nurturing to rough-housing and teaching the children about money management. Marlene enjoyed parenting more than she'd imagined she would, and saw Paul as a fully participating father. Their marital bond reinforced their parental bond. They had worries about parenting during adolescence, but viewed these as challenges.

Not all couples can develop and implement equity guidelines as successfully as Marlene and Paul, yet the equity model is relevant to most marriages.

As a couple approaches their fortieth birthdays, new issues arise. By then they have probably been married between ten and fifteen years. If they are going to make major changes in their lives or marriages, this is the time to do so. Some couples find this period particularly rocky, and consider separation or divorce. Often the issue is that the woman is growing more independent and assertive, and becoming more involved in her career or community organizations. At the same time, the man has risen to a certain level in his career and is now more interested in devoting time and energy to his wife and family. Many couples find that their personal interests and goals are no longer complementary. This can lead to misunderstanding, conflict, and emotional distance, as well as their feeling unappreciated and unloved.

Ann and Ken. This couple was feeling good about their mutual growth and development, at least until Ken was forty-three and Ann forty-one. In their early thirties, after the birth of their second child they had experienced stress and sought marital therapy. They had remained in therapy for over a year, exploring feelings, learning communication techniques, identifying destructive patterns learned from observing their parents' marriages. and discussing personal development within the marriage. More recently they had entered a marital enrichment program sponsored by their church. Ken and Ann were considered by many to be an ideal couple.

When their children grew older, Ann had returned to school and completed a Masters degree. She had been working full time for three years; in the past two she'd been promoted twice. She found herself bringing home a great deal of work, and was traveling on a regular basis. Ken had reached a middle-management position in which he felt stable and secure, although not particularly satisfied. Over the past five years, he had consciously moderated his work load and drastically reduced his out-of-town travel. He became more active around the home and coached his son's baseball team. Clearly they were at different places in their interests: Ann putting a lot of herself into her career, Ken wanting to emphasize home and family. Ken's changes were in response to Ann's request that he not be so work- and performance-oriented, and he resented her doing now what he had done ten years before. She was less available to share companionship, parent the children, and be an energetic sex partner. He felt cheated and resentful and reacted by distancing himself. Ann was feeling a combination of exhilaration and guilt. She enjoyed her career, her feelings of competence, and friendships with colleagues. Yet she worried that the children and Ken were feeling slighted. She resented that becoming more her own person meant she had to deal with feelings of guilt and pressure from her husband and family.

For six months their marriage endured a painful, emotional period dominated by resentment. They were no longer the ideal couple they'd been although they continued to participate in couple activities, which helped them through this difficult transitional period. Especially helpful was a regular sex life and the pleasure of family activities. Their marriage was able to survive these personal changes while maintaining the essential emotional and sexual bond.

There were no simple solutions for Ken and Ann. They needed to state their desires, plans, and fears clearly, to listen without being defensive, and to negotiate agreements. Ann wanted to be rid of guilty feelings. Ken agreed to cease critical comments as long as Ann was honest with him about her plans and time constraints. Ann realized that when she made promises she couldn't keep Ken got angry, and she felt guilty. Ken came to accept that his involvement with the children and his other activities were in his best interest, and that he was not doing them to placate Ann. His desire for her to return to their previous lifestyle was recognized as unrealistic and inappropriate. Couples have to live their lives as they now exist; they can't turn the clock back.

Ann and Ken are a good example of a couple whose marriage survived because they were aware of conflicts and willing to deal with them. Good marriages are not devoid of conflict, pain, and disappointment. Good marriages are characterized by sharing both happy and sad experiences, by a commitment to dealing with individual and couple issues, and the ability to grow as people and as a couple.

CLOSING THOUGHTS

The equity model of marriage involves the couple's having freedom for individual development while maintaining a sense of couple growth and intimacy. They are aware of the stresses and tensions that occur as a result of balancing careers, children, and a changing sexual relationship. They recognize that there are more similarities than differences between women and men. They value empathy, respect, trust, and intimacy, and strive to nurture their couple bond. Just as important, they are committed to problem solving and reaching mutually satisfying agreements. A satisfying and stable marriage brings out the best in each individual, involves a positive influence process, and is based on respect and equity.

6

GUIDELINES FOR YOUR MARITAL AND SEXUAL RELATIONSHIP

There are no rigid right and wrong rules applicable to all marriages. Each couple needs to develop their unique marital and sexual style. These guidelines can increase your awareness and help make your marriage more satisfying and secure. We believe in these guidelines theoretically, utilize them clinically, and try to apply them personally.

1. The more intimate your relationship, the better the sex.
2. The better the communication, especially the ability to make clear and direct sexual requests, the more satisfying your sexual relationship.
3. Setting aside couple time is crucial to keep your intimate relationship satisfying.
4. Affection and touching should occur in the regular course of your life, both inside and outside the bedroom.
5. Be spontaneous and playful in your sexual interactions.
6. Maintain an attitude of sexual experimentation and openness.
7. Learn to laugh off, or at least not overreact to, medicore unsatisfying sexual experiences.
8. Both men and women can enjoy pleasuring/foreplay, intercourse, and afterplay.

9. Understand and accept changes in sexual response and body image that come with the maturing of the relationship and the aging process.

10. Maintain an attitude of caring and commitment which nurtures the marital bond.

Let's consider each guideline as specifically and explicitly as possible. Sometimes couples attempt to apply techniques that experts say will improve their marriage, and find that not only don't they help, but they're actually harmful. For certain marriages, a particular guideline is simply not appropriate. More often, although your intention might be good and you're using the "right" terminology, your emotional and behavioral follow-through in applying the guideline is weak. We have listened with amazement to couples who claimed to be communicating honestly, but instead were being defensive and manipulative; couples who said they argued well but were intimidating and hitting below the belt; couples supposedly having fun together who actually were having a dull time doing something neither really wanted to because it was the "in" thing, couples who claimed open, experimental, and playful sexual interactions in which one partner made demands and pushed the other to engage in stimulation techniques he didn't want.

These ten guidelines are complex attitudes and skills that require practice, clear and constructive feedback, and refinement before they become a comfortable part of your couple style. Reading and making a New Year's resolution to change is not enough. Thought and psychological energy are required as well as the commitment to work on these guidelines and talk about how to implement them.

Guideline 1. The more intimate your relationship, the better the sex.

There is an age-old theoretical argument, "Can you have sex without love?" Of course you can. People can be sexually functional in nonloving relationships; the scientific data on that question is clear. However psychologists, marriage therapists, and sex therapists believe that sexuality is most satisfying in the context of an intimate, committed relationship. Emotional intimacy involves revealing yourself to your spouse—not only your loving feelings and positive characteristics, but also weaknesses and doubts about yourself. In an intimate marriage, you have the freedom to reveal them and still be loved and accepted. You don't need to maintain secrets, or worry that if your spouse knew them she would not love or respect you. Intimacy means sharing not only happy, loving feelings but also problems, disappointments, and angry feelings. These can be dealt with in the context of an intimate, secure marriage. You trust your spouse not to abuse your disclosures, to support you through bad times, and to accept problem areas and not use them against you. Your spouse respects and loves you for who you really are, not the public image you project.

Sexually, you can enjoy giving and receiving pleasure *with* each other rather than needing to perform *for* each other. If you are not lubricated or do not have an erection, your partner will not berate you but will accept that this is a bad time for sexual intercourse. You could engage in sensual touching or a nonintercourse sexual scenario. Your couple style can allow both partners to initiate and request a range of sensual and sexual activities. If you want to be the receiver of cunnilingus or fellatio and not have to reciprocate this time, your spouse can enjoy giving you pleasure without saying, "Now you owe me one." Intimacy is *not* idealized romantic and problem-free sexuality. Being intimate includes giving and receiving negative feedback and dealing with problem situations. It means listening to the partner when she says she wants him to talk more just before he has an orgasm, or when he tells her to touch his penis more firmly and stroke it with a faster rhythm. Intimacy means sharing sexual desires, feelings, and requests as you experience them at the time—the key to creative sexuality.

Guideline 2. The better the communication, especially the ability to make clear and direct sexual requests, the more satisfying your sexual relationship.

Communication is both one of the most crucially important and one of the most poorly used concepts in human behavior. We are advocating personal, clear, direct, and high-quality communication. This is very different from the general, ambiguous, indirect, and low-quality communication that is typical of many. It is the difference between saying, "What would you like to do?" or "I want you to massage me just the way I tell you or I won't get turned on," and saying, "I like the way you're stroking me, but I'd enjoy it if you moved your hand about an inch and touched in a gentler, more tender way." Communication can and should be both verbal and nonverbal. The ability to guide your partner by putting your hand over his and showing where and how you wish to be touched is an excellent skill to develop. This "hand override" technique is very effective nonverbal sexual communication. Another nonverbal method of requesting is to take your partner's hand or head and move it to the area you want him to stimulate.

It's vital to be aware of the difference between a request and a demand. A request is *asking* something from your spouse. You state your feelings as clearly as you can, and what you want, as well as your concern for his perceptions and feelings. Your partner can accept the request, reject it, or modify it, depending on his desires. A demand says he must do it now, do it your way, or there will be consequences. Requests result in sharing pleasure, demands result in feelings of anger, resentment, and pressure to meet performance requirements. Requests are a communication which enhances the couple bond. Demands allow you to get what you want at the moment, but cause breaches in communication and the relationships. With requests, opportunities for emotional and sexual intimacy are broadened.

Guideline 3. Setting aside couple time is crucial to keep your intimate relationship satisfying.

This is the most important guideline. We, like many couples, live hectic lives with demands on our time from children, careers, household chores, friends, and community activities. Our couple time receives a high priority; it is jealousy guarded.

Couple time might consist of a fifteen-minute chat on the porch, drinking tea and sharing our experiences and feelings about the week, dinner together, without the kids or friends, and then a long walk, or a weekend trip to the city—as a couple, not as a family. While doing chores separately at home, you could make a date to meet over a drink at ten that night and discuss what you've been doing, chat about the next day, or engage in touching or caressing that may or may not proceed to intercourse. It is easy to take your spouse for granted and allow the couple bond to gradually erode. Couples say they have time together because they see each other coming and going. The couple time we're advocating is quality interactive time. It involves touching and talking in which you connect emotionally and feel cared about.

Couple time includes the period before and after intercourse. Getting out of a relaxing bath—during which your spouse has come in and out of the bathroom talking and teasing—and, as you dry off, receiving an invitation to come to bed can be exciting. The afterplay experience is a particularly good time to be together and talk. After sharing sex, it is easier and natural to share feelings about you as an individual and couple. People are more emotionally open and vulnerable before and after a sexual experience.

Guideline 4. Affection and touching should occur in the regular course of your life, both inside and outside the bedroom.

Pleasure and affection belong in your life, not just in the bedroom when the lights are out, the kids asleep, and his penis is in her vagina. Many couples feel they have outgrown the stage where they hold hands and really kiss (not the perfunctory peck on the cheek). That's a destructive myth; you never outgrow your need for touching and affection. Maintaining affectionate contact as a regular part of your life allows sexual feelings to flow naturally rather than isolating sex as an activity unto itself, separate from the rest of your life.

It's fun to stimulate your partner's breast as she's bending over to kiss you goodbye on her way to work in the morning. The pleasant images from that interaction linger throughout the day and make it more likely you'll feel sexual in the evening.

A hug and kiss while paying bills is comforting. Having extra contact and support while doing one of life's most odious tasks makes it more livable. Being affectionate while watching TV with the kids in the family room can be good for both you and the children. Seeing parents touching, hugging, and kissing is a good model for children. We are not suggesting being sensual or sexual in front of the children—that is a private activity. However, being affectionate in front of the children, or having family hugs, is a positive part of sexuality education. Integrating touching and affection in your life—whether in the kitchen or bedroom, in your car or walking in public, as a couple or in front of the children—is an affirmation of your caring for each other and a source of sexual desire. Sexuality is more than genitals, intercourse, and the few seconds of orgasm. Sexuality is a way of expressing warmth, affection, attraction, sensuality, and desire.

Guideline 5. Be spontaneous and playful in your sexual interactions.

Sex is particularly nice when it's tender and warm, and extends over a two-hour period. It can have all the romance of a candlelight dinner with wine, lobster, and intercourse as dessert. However, if that were the format for each sexual experience, it would become dull, routine, and predictable. It's nice to spice up life with a "quickie" or stand-up intercourse; sometimes you need tuna salad or hamburger so you can appreciate steak. When you're in touch with your desires and feelings, your sexual experiences will be more spontaneous and creative. Spontaneous, unplanned sex can be as satisfying as planned, romantic sex. Sometimes sex can be intense and passionate, other times tender and sensuous. Waking up before your partner and waking him by stroking his penis can be arousing, but so can being warm, slow, and sensuous. The key is to be aware of your feelings and open to your spouse's feelings.

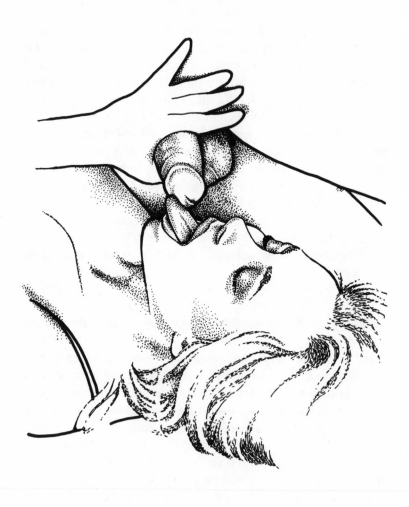

The mouth and genitals are the most pleasure-giving and pleasure receiving parts of the human body. Oral sex is intimate, pleasurable and satisfying for the giver and the receiver.

Sexual arousal can arise from being silly and playful. For example, while playing cards and joking, you could have a simulated fight with a resulting desire for sex. If you're a couple who are usually task-oriented in the morning, go back to bed on a whim after breakfast. After a hard game of tennis, take a shower and engage in a second game—of sex! Playfulness need not always result in sexual intercourse. Enjoy the playful or sensual moment for itself. Those times it does lead to intercourse are all the better.

Guideline 6. Maintain an attitude of sexual experimentation and openness.

If you believe you know all there is to know about each other sexually and that there is no need for further experimentation, this becomes a self-fulfilling prophecy and there is no further sharing or learning. The resulting marital sex is dull, routine, and stagnant. You start feeling that the only way to spice up your sex life is to have an affair. When your attitude is one of experimentation and openness, then it too becomes a self-fulfilling prophecy, and marital sex continues to evolve and remain satisfying.

We have been married over twenty-three years, and never cease to be amazed at new sexual awareness about ourselves, each other, and how we as a couple can share pleasure. In large part this comes from our conscious commitment to experiment and learn sexually. When we first married, we believed that the hard task would be to develop an open, expressive sexual style. What we have come to understand is that the real challenge is to commit the time and energy to maintain a satisfying marital and sexual bond.

We set aside time for a more open and extended sexual session every six weeks or so. The focus is experimenting with something new. We might do something simple, such as using a new body lotion or trying a variation of an intercourse position. Other times we might be more elaborate, like going to an old inn and, after a candlelight dinner, making love on an eighteenth-century couch. Or we drop the children at a baby sitter and return home, take the phone off the hook, and have a three-hour love session in the family room in front of the fireplace listening to a new tape we've bought for the occasion. Other couples use techniques such as pretending they're on a first date and engaging in the coy give-and-take of the sexual seduction game. Experiment with what fits your feelings and needs. Attitude is the key—the awareness of and desire to continue experimenting, learning, and growing. You care enough about your marriage and sex in your marriage to keep it open and satisfying.

Guideline 7. Learn to laugh off, or at least not overreact, mediocre or unsatisfying sexual experiences.

An oppressive new sex myth is the belief that all sexual experiences should be fully functional and equally arousing for both partners. Otherwise, according to this myth, you have a sexual dysfunction or hang-up. In reality, couples who report a high level of satisfaction with their sexual lives indicate that about 40 percent of their sexual experiences are very satisfactory for both partners; about 30 percent of the time one partner finds it very fulfilling, while the other finds it enjoyable; about 20 percent of sexual interactions are moderately satisfying for one partner, and the other has relatively little feeling (although perhaps enjoying the response of the spouse); and in approximately 5 to 10 percent of sexual interactions, sex is either mediocre or simply does not work. This happens with us, as it does to other couples. Somewhere in the middle of pleasuring or even during intercourse, one of us—usually Barry—will ask if the other is "into it." If the response is, "No, but I thought you were," we'll laugh it off and say, "Let's be sexual tomorrow night." We try to get together in the next day or two so that thoughts of the unsatisfying sexual experience don't linger.

Many couples overreact to a poor sexual experience and either don't talk about it or endlessly discuss the problem and whose fault it was. If mediocre sex is a frequent occurrence, you need to discuss your couple sexual style in an open and frank manner. However, if it is infrequent, accept sexual response as variable and don't make it a major issue. To use a cliché, don't make a mountain out of a molehill. Mediocre, uninteresting, or "failed," sexual experiences are not only to be expected, but are a natural aspect of your humanness and variability as a couple. You don't always cook a perfect dinner or have a wonderful time at a party, nor do your children always behave perfectly. It is unrealistic to expect your sex to be always satisfying. There is a next time, and that time will be easier if this time you can laugh and be accepting.

Guideline 8. Both men and women can enjoy pleasuring/ foreplay, intercourse, and afterplay.

Many couples consider pleasuring/foreplay to be primarily or exclusively to ready the woman for intercourse. A "sophisticated" man considers foreplay not as a duty but as a mark of concern for his wife and a measure of his expertise as a lover. The idea that a man can enjoy sensuality and pleasuring strikes him as unmasculine. In the same manner, intercourse is viewed as the domain of the male, although there is pressure on women to have an orgasm during intercourse. Of course, once a man ejaculates sex is over, so you might as well roll over and go to sleep. These rigid perceptions of the sexual scenario cause miscommunication and resentment. They build performance anxiety, reduce the sense of pleasure, and interfere with the couple's becoming a sexual team.

Pleasuring/foreplay, intercourse, and afterplay are integral expressions of sexuality rather than arbitrary components in which the male takes one role and the female another. Pleasure is open to both partners throughout the sexual experience. Female sexual response is more *complex* and *variable* than male sexual response. For most women, arousal takes longer and requires more time spent setting the mood, engaging in nongenital pleasuring, and direct genital stimulation. The woman might be nonorgasmic, singly orgasmic, or multiorgasmic, which can occur during pleasuring, intercourse, or afterplay. The male typically has one orgasm. Female sexual response is different, not better or worse, than male response. Sexuality is a matter of pleasure and mutuality, not of performance and competition.

Both can enjoy pleasuring. This is unlikely to happen if the man "does the woman" for twenty minutes with the sole goal of arousing her so that she is ready for intercourse. Sex is more involving and arousing if there is mutual pleasuring. Sexuality is more satisfying when there is openness to giving and receiving pleasure-oriented touching. The male needs to be aware that he can enjoy slow, teasing arousal during which his erection might wax and wane. He can be open to receiving as well as giving pleasure. The slower, more interactive pleasuring scenario results in more satisfying intercourse and orgasm.

As you share pleasure in the process of mutual arousal and stop seeing it as work toward a goal, intercourse can be viewed as a natural extension of mutual pleasuring. Sex is not an act in which the male must respond with an erection and the female must respond with an orgasm. Some women are orgasmic with intercourse. Most women enjoy intercourse, but find it easier and more pleasurable to be orgasmic with manual, oral, or rubbing stimulation. This is a matter of couple style and preference, not a question of a "right" or "wrong" way to have an orgasm. Intercourse is a close, intimate sharing and coming together. It is not necessary for the woman to be orgasmic during intercourse to meet her partner's expectations or to prove something to herself or anyone else. Intercourse will be more satisfying for both people if they focus on mutual enjoyment and pleasure and not on erectile or orgasmic performance. Intercourse is best viewed as a natural extension of the pleasuring process, not apart from that process.

The afterplay period is not just tacked on; it is an integral part of lovemaking. Physiologically, you have just shared an intense experience and your body returns gradually to the unstimulated state. Psychologically, this is an excellent time to share feelings and touching. Some couples enjoy lying together and holding each other; others will drink a glass of wine and talk; still others might engage in a playful pillow fight. The important thing is that afterplay involves mutual sharing and pleasure.

Guideline 9. Understand and accept changes in sexual response and body image that come with the maturing of the relationship and the aging process.

Our bodies change gradually in both appearance and function as we age. Aging does not mean becoming nonsexual, unless you fall into the trap of narrowly defining your sexuality on youth, beauty, and rapid response. The couple who view sexuality as pleasure-oriented, who realize that arousal can come from sharing and stimulation, and who enjoy the receptivity and responsivity of their partner, will find sex satisfying as they age. The changes that occur with aging are gradual, not drastic. Aging alters your sexual functioning but does not end it. You are a sexual person from the day you're born to the day you die.

Your self-image and sexual response are influenced by how you treat yourself. If you gain weight, do not exercise, smoke, drink to excess, and do not attend to your body, you will feel less physically good and less sexually responsive. People who take care of their bodies, have regular sleep patterns, eat heathily, exercise, do not smoke, and drink moderately are more likely to be physically healthy and sexually responsive.

As you age, sexual arousal is slower and the need for a continuous sexual outlet lessens, but the enjoyment of being together and experiencing pleasure, arousal, and orgasm is very much there. Men no longer function automatically and autonomously, and that can be an advantage for the couple. Sharing, interactive sexuality is superior to automatic arousal and erections. Youthful sex is like a wild, exciting ride over unexplored rapids, with excitement from the sense of conquest and unexpected adventure. Mature sex is like skillfully canoeing a scenic river that you've explored and learned to enjoy, and can savor its changing moods and seasons. The couple who accept their aging as a natural evolution and not a tragic event have a self-enhancing attitude that will deliver continual sexual dividends.

Guideline 10. Maintain an attitude of caring and commitment which nurtures the marital bond.

When a couple begins dating, they experience romantic ecstasy. There is a sense of novelty, an excitement about what will develop, and a willingness to overcome barriers in order to be with your lover. Some feel it is tragic that romantic ecstasy does not last. We believe it is a good thing. Marriage cannot be based on novelty, ecstasy, and conquest. Seeking a perpetual return to these states is self-defeating and leads to frustration because your expectations will be consistently thwarted. Going backward only works in the movies. Emotional and sexual intimacy form a more mature, solid, and secure basis for marital sex. With these it is possible—and indeed critical—for you as a couple to grow while maintaining a commitment to the marital bond. Changing involves an integration of the old and new. You change as you age and your life situation changes. Part of the couple commitment is to be aware of those changes and their effects on your marital relationship.

If you read about an oral sex technique you'd like to experiment with, request it in a caring way and refrain from being demanding. The style in which you adapt the oral sex experience may be diffrent from that described in the book. Don't worry about keeping up with new sexual trends. Be aware of your past experiences and preferences, and choose how to integrate new techniques and scenarios into your lovemaking.

Growing entails an attitude that you can change as an individual rather than stagnating, and that these changes can be integrated into your couple bond. In marriage, there will be periods of stress, frustration, and discomfort. There will also be periods of joy, discovery, and pride. Dealing with a difficult situation and solving a problem strengthens the couple bond. Learning that you can cope with problems is a stressful but growing experience. Sharing sad as well as joyful experiences increases intimate feelings. A satisfying, intimate, and secure marriage entails being open to sexual and emotional growth, dealing with both the good and the bad.

CLOSING THOUGHTS

These guidelines are to help you think and talk about sexuality within your marriage and what you can do to optimize marital sex. They are not hard-and-fast rules set in concrete. Apply these guidelines so they are helpful in developing your marital and sexual style. The guidelines emphasize enhancing attitudes even more than specific behavior. You owe it yourself and your marriage to grow as individuals and as a couple.

7
SEXUAL VARIATIONS:
WHEN DOES EXPERIMENTATION
BECOME KINKY?

Variety and experimentation are catchwords used by popular writers as well as marriage and sex therapists. But what do they mean? Learning to be comfortable with giving and receiving oral sex? Or becoming involved in swinging and group ambisexuality? If we as a couple choose to experiment sexually and break out of our inhibited patterns, do we have to go all the way and try everything we've heard or read about? Do we need to *prove* we're liberated?

Variety and experimentation are healthy for marital sexuality. We encourage couples to experiment with a wide variety of sexual techniques and scenarios, within certain guidelines. Experimentation should *not* be to prove anything to anyone, nor should it involve performance demands or be manipulative or coercive. Experimentation can be nondemanding, with the intent of increased sharing and pleasure. As long as the focus is on pleasure and not performance, on requests rather than demands, on honesty and not manipulation, experimentation can enhance sexuality. If you approach it as mutual exploration you will not feel disappointed or intimidated. You are not on a search for a goal, but on a journey during which you enjoy the sexual discovery process. Be open to experiences that enhance sexual expression.

Before setting out on this journey, allow us to offer a warning: don't fall into the new, sexually sophisticated trap of feeling you have to prove you are sexually liberated. The notion that you "should" desire each new sexual technique—whether anal stimulation, being sexual in a hot tub, masturbating in front of your partner, watching X-rated movies, making love standing up, or having group sex fantasies—is just another form of sexual fascism. Being sexually comfortable and free means accepting your sexual preferences and choices as a sexual person and couple. Couples who feel that they must try each sexual technique in order to prove they are not inhibited are in a worse position than sexually repressed couples. With this in mind, let us examine some sexual variations and scenarios.

ORAL SEX

The mouth and genitals are the two most pleasure-giving and pleasure-receiving parts of the human body. Traditionally, oral-genital sex has been viewed as exotic and exciting, but also anxiety-provoking and guilt-inducing. Oral sex is not only normal but one of the most intimate, pleasurable, and satisfying means of expressing yourself with the person you love. As with any sexual technique, there will be individual differences and preferences in its use. Those individuals or couples who choose not to engage in or who do not enjoy oral-genital stimulation are normal, not sexually repressed. It is your right and choice not to include oral sex in your repertoire.

It is interesting but baffling why so much of oral sexual behavior (cunnilingus and fellatio) is shrouded in a cloud of dirtiness, or at least naughtiness. Slang terms such as "go down on," "69", "blow job," "eat her out," and "suck him off" have negative, and often aggressive, connotations. In pornographic magazines and X-rated movies, there is an inordinate emphasis on oral-genital sex, with special emphasis on domination and humiliation. The subtle—and not so subtle—message is that oral sex is exciting but degrading, an act of lust rather than one of pleasure, passion, and intimacy. The perception is that oral sex is primarily for men. The woman's role is to pretend she enjoys it. The joke is that men are on the lookout for a

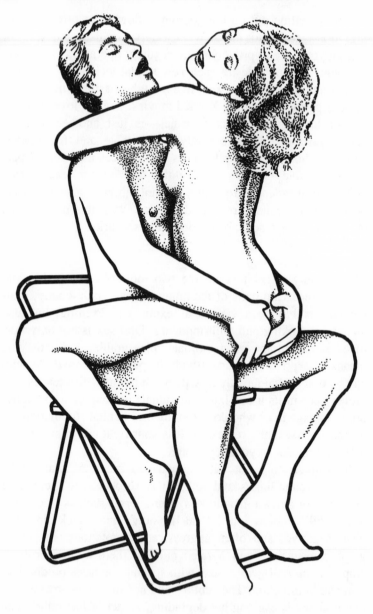

Intercourse in the sitting position allows you to experience alternate ways of making love.

woman who is willing to let him ejaculate in her mouth (and swallow his semen), but she's perverted if she does.

The truth is that oral sex is pleasurable and loving, a way of sharing yourself intimately without connotations of dominance or humiliation. You can enjoy high levels of arousal and lusty feelings without concern that you're perverse or animalistic. Both women and men can enjoy giving and receiving oral stimulation.

What are the best oral-genital techniques? Is it okay if he ejaculates in her mouth? What if she passes gas while he's orally stimulating her? Is it acceptable if he thrusts his pelvis or should he be passive? Why does she feel self-conscious when he's lying between her legs? Why is it easier for her to be multiorgasmic when he's performing cunnilingus? Is mutual oral sex ("69") better than taking turns? Is the taste of vaginal secretions bad for his breath? These are among the questions couples have but are too embarrassed to ask and share with each other. There is no one best technique nor one right way to engage in oral sex. We will present guidelines, address the most common questions, and encourage you to experiment, share, and choose your preferences and style.

The best way to approach oral-genital sex is comfortably. Oral sex can involve kissing, licking, sucking, biting. Start by doing oral stimulation on other body parts—neck, back, breasts, face—before moving to the genitals. Try stimulation with one partner giving to the other before going on to mutual oral stimulation. Instead of demanding or pressing for orgasm, focus on nondemand oral-genital pleasuring first. Explore and see what feels good and what your partner enjoys. Most people are not responsive to oral stimulation unless they are moderately aroused. He might run his tongue around her vulva before doing a rapid sucking motion focused on the inner lips and clitoral area. Oral stimulation, like manual and intercourse stimulation, progresses from slower, more tender touching. This allows the arousal process to gradually build to more intense, erotic stimulation.

For many women, oral stimulation is the easiest and fastest way to achieve arousal and orgasm. More women experience

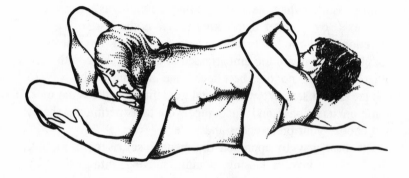

Many couples find mutual oral-genital sex the most arousing kind of multiple stimulation. Each can let go and express their passion.

multiorgasmic response with cunnilingus than with any other sexual technique. Although males feel highly aroused through oral stimulation, they may be embarrassed or self-conscious asking for or directing the partner in what is most pleasurable. The woman therefore feels confused, because she experiences pressure to orally stimulate his penis but has no guidance or feedback about what to do. As is true of other sexual techniques, oral sex does not come naturally. Even basics, such as putting the penis to the side of the mouth so it doesn't cause a gag reflex or holding your hand on his penis while he thrusts, need to be communicated about and practiced. Start oral stimulation by kissing or licking around the shaft of the penis before putting it in your mouth. Do what's comfortable for you—stimulating the glans with your tongue, sucking with your lips closed, moving your tongue around when the penis is in your mouth—before asking what's best for him.

The question of his ejaculation is one of the most emotionally loaded and individualistic preferences. Does he want to? Some men prefer oral sex for arousal and ejaculate only during intercourse. Others not only want to ejaculate, but see it as symbolic that she swallow the semen. Semen is germfree, safe, and even has low caloric content. Many women do not like semen gushing into their mouths, and so can enjoy sucking and licking the penis, but not ejaculation. The couple have to establish, in a noncoercive manner, a style of oral sex that allows comfort and pleasure for each. The most common pattern is to use fellatio as a pleasuring technique and then switch to intercourse. When fellatio is pursued to orgasm, the male usually withdraws right before he ejaculates.

WEEKENDS AWAY

Are parents selfish, hedonistic people if they enjoy weekends away without the children? Is your life an endless seeking of excitement and relief without attending to responsibilities and caring for your children? Should you feel guilty about taking time for yourselves as a couple, especially when sexual sharing is a major component of the enjoyment?

We firmly believe weekends away without children is one of the best things you can do for yourself and your marriage. The central relationship in a family is the husband-wife bond. As long as this remains strong, it is easier to deal with career, financial, extended family, home, and child-rearing issues. We try to have at least one and preferably two weekends a year to ourselves to reenergize our couple bond.

Sex is not the most important aspect of marriage, but it is integral to the couple bond. Sexuality has three important functions—sharing a pleasurable experience, reducing tension, and reinforcing emotional and sexual intimacy. A weekend away allows time and privacy to be a sexual couple. The strengthened couple bond allows you to function better as a person and a parent, around the house and in your job.

When our children were younger, we traded babysitting with other families and watched their children when they took a weekend away. Our children looked forward to this because it gave them a chance to have their friends spend a whole weekend. Believe it or not, it's not that much harder to watch six rather than three children; they entertain and take care of each other.

Your weekend away need not be focused on sex. You can enjoy skiing, sailing, seeing a play, antiquing, reading a book, sightseeing, and going to dinner. However, do not overschedule. Be sure you have time for each other, to talk and for leisurely sex. Being together, holding hands, and touching can build a sensual mood. Weekends away allow experimentation with sex in the morning, afternoon, or early evening. Break out of the "sex as the last thing at night after everything else is taken care of" routine.

It is important to have weekends away when your children are young. The parent of a young child knows how easy it is for children to dominate your every waking moment. What is less apparent is the need to have weekends away when the children are older, especially during adolescence. Adolescence can be a tumultuous and difficult time. Not surprisingly, one of the most stressful periods in adult life is parenting adolescents. You need a weekend away to reenergize you and your marital bond. It also helps to prepare you for the stage of being a couple again when children have left home.

One of our favorite pleasures was to return to our house and spend a weekend at home without the children and with the answering machine on. Whatever you do and however you as a couple decide to do it, a weekend or even a night away is a way to revitalize yourself, your relationship, and your sexuality. It can be a creative time. Many of the ideas for this book were developed on our weekends away.

NONDEMAND SENSUALITY

Whoever heard of a married couple being playful, sexually teasing, and not proceeding to intercourse? Being nude and having a sensual body massage just to enjoy the experience? Being aroused, and maybe orgasmic, but choosing not to engage in intercourse? A perversion? No, it is a way to keep in touch with your sensuality and sexuality. To reaffirm sexuality as a way to share pleasure and intimacy, not a command performance. Touching and being sensual without the demand that it culminate in intercourse each time is one of the best ways to keep a relationship fresh and spontaneous. It has the beneficial side effect of increasing intercourse frequency. Since you keep physical contact, when one or the other feels aroused and desirous of intercourse, the transition from touching to intercourse is easier.

We set aside an evening about once every six weeks to engage in a variety of nondemand pleasuring experiences, agreeing beforehand that they will *not* end in intercourse. Sometimes the evening is a relaxing one during which we lie around, drink wine, and listen to music. The touching will be gentle and sensuous, but not erotic. At other times, sexual arousal will build during the night, as the teasing touching and sensuality increases anticipation and results in erotic feelings that may proceed to orgasm for one or both, depending on our feelings and desires. This brings back memories of teenage years, when petting and necking were particularly exciting, before we engage in the "real thing." Couples have the attitude that since intercourse is permissible, enjoyment of anticipation, uncertainty, and arousal is no longer acceptable. Touching that does not proceed to intercourse is derogatorily labeled "immature" or "sexual teasing." What nonsense. This attitude is a major reason for mechanical, routine, and unsatisfying marital sex. Part of the excitement of the teenage years was that sex was filled with a sense of adventure, exploration, and unpredictability. Now it is easy to fall into the trap of pleasuring always leading to—planned and expected intercourse. Pleasuring can add excitement, variety, and a sense of exploration, spontaneity, and unpredictability to your sex life. Nondemand sensuality is a prime source of sexual desire.

MASTURBATION

Did you know that well over half of married women and men occasionally masturbate? The old view of masturbation is that it was a form of self-abuse which caused all kinds of physical and psychological problems, from acne to social isolation. A recent, more enlightened view was that masturbation was a developmental phase that young men—but not women, heaven forbid! —experienced, which ceased after they began having intercourse. Recent research and clinical practice indicates that masturbation is the best way for a man or woman to learn about his or her body, sexual responsivity, and orgasmic pattern. Both men and women masturbate before marriage, and both masturbate after marriage. In fact, rates of female masturbation increase after marriage.

For the married person, masturbation can serve many functions. It can be a way of dealing with sexual desires when the partner is away or ill; it can provide a mechanism to keep in touch with your sexuality or serve as an orgasmic outlet when there is a discrepancy in partners' sex drives, or be a vehicle to experiment with a new pleasuring technique or fantasy. Of course, as with all aspects of sexuality, masturbation can be misused. Masturbation can be employed as a weapon to make your spouse uncomfortable, a way to avoid dealing with sexual dissatisfaction, or as a means of keeping emotional and sexual distance.

One exercise employed in sex therapy is masturbation in front of the partner. This can be arousing, especially for the person observing. It provides an excellent way to teach your partner how you like to be touched and your pattern of sexual arousal. Consider whether this form of experimentation would be worthwhile for you.

DIFFERENT SETTINGS AND TIMES

For most couples, sex = the bedroom late at night. Couples say sex is important, but it is given the last priority in their life—late at night, when all other important and unimportant chores have been completed. What about setting aside a different time and place for a sexual encounter? Physiologically, the best time for sex is in the morning. Your body is rested, sleep and dreams have rested your mind, and testosterone levels in men are highest in the morning. On weekends, rather than jumping out of bed to start chores, or getting the paper and busily informing yourself of all the world's woes, why not take time to be sensual and/or sexual? Waking up to a gentle massage, having your breasts fondled or your penis stroked, is better than a cup of coffee. You might like a "quickie" intercourse before leaving for work. You could carry pleasant sexual memories during the day, with a feeling that the evening will be more romantic and mutually involving.

What about nooners? Instead of a long business lunch at which you eat too much, drink too much, and spend too much money, come home and add a little sexual pleasure to your day. During the weekend, ask your neighbors to watch your children or get the kids involved in some activity so that you can go upstairs, lock the door, take the phone off the hook, and enjoy yourself.

What about sex before dinner or early in the evening? Exercise—including sex—before eating improves digestive processes. If you can't sleep, or you wake early, what about occasionally waking your partner by fondling and caressing?

Nothing is more unexpected than to be waking up slowly and realizing that your partner is aroused and desires you.

What would it be like to make love in your kitchen? On the rug in front of the fireplace? What about a deserted beach, or in the back seat of the car like you did twenty years before? Of course, the bedroom is more convenient and comfortable, but at times wouldn't you like to be adventuresome and take some risks? Even more intriguing, what about going to your office at night or on a weekend when no one is there? You could have sex in your office chair, on the rug, or even on the desk— pleasant memories for when you're stuck in a boring business meeting or having a hard time with a report. In suggesting these, we don't want you to feel pressured to do any or all, but to consider whether you want to try one or two on for size and see if they fit your marital needs.

SEXUAL FANTASIES

Sexual fantasies are the most flexible and adaptable aphrodisiacs. People use fantasies during masturbation and feel fine about it. However, people feel strange using fantasies when having sex with their spouses. Does it mean she wants to be unfaithful?

The great majority of us have unusual and even bizarre sexual fantasies at least occasionally. You might fantasize about forced sex or being forced, friends watching and admiring your sexual performance, five people trying to make love to you at the same time, or having a ménage-à-trois with your spouse and business partner. These fantasies are hard to accept, but the hardest of all, although the most frequent, are fantasies about another partner. Whether it's the next door neighbor, the person at the drugstore, your spouse's best friend, an attractive individual you see on the bus, or a movie star, you feel anxious or guilty. This is especially true when you're fantasizing about having sex with someone else during intercourse with your spouse.

Having and enjoying a fantasy is not the same thing as desiring to actually experience the behavior. Most of us would not like, much less participate in, the sex fantasies we use. A characteristic of fantasies that gives them special power and pull is that they are illicit, have socially unacceptable themes, and rebel against societal norms. It is one thing to enjoy the image; it is altogether different to act out the behavior.

Most fantasies are best kept as fantasies. When people do try to act them out, they are usually disappointed and get into situations that can have bad consequences. Fantasizing about sex with someone else is natural and harmless. Don't view it as a sign of unfaithfulness or as meaning that you don't want to be making love with your intimate partner. You are having sex with each other and enjoying it—including the fantasies. The role of fantasy is to spice up your sex life. Fantasies are best thought of as an additional stimulation technique that builds a bridge to greater sexual arousal. They will only get you into trouble when they become obsessive or associated with guilt. Give yourself permission to use a range of fantasies to enhance sexual desire.

The next techniques are four that we ourselves choose not to engage in, but this is a question of preference. Don't judge a technique as "normal" or "abnormal." As long as the two of you agree to try it, and don't feel coerced, are not trying to prove something, and it isn't done in a harmful or compulsive manner, it is a variant of sexual expression. You might choose to try it experimentally or just occasionally, or it may become an important part of your couple sexual style.

VIBRATORS

In our technological society, where everything else is being done by machines, shouldn't we at least keep sex natural? Do we need mechanical gadgets to make us aroused and orgasmic? No, we don't *need* them, but many couples find that a vibrator can add variety to lovemaking and enhance sexual responsiveness.

Vibrators first came into widespread use as an adjunct to female masturbation. Although there are many different types of vibrators, the most popular are hand-held, battery-operated, two-speed models with two to four attachments. They are sold

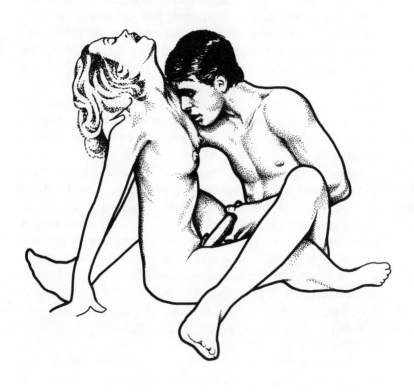

Vibrator stimulation can enhance arousal before or during intercourse.

in drug or department stores as hand, face, or back massagers as well as in sex shops.

Couples who report deriving the most pleasure from vibrators are those who use them as an adjunct to touching, not as a magic toy that substitutes for partner contact. Some couples use a vibrator solely as a means of enhancing a sensual massage. Others will use the vibrator to increase sexual arousal before intercourse. Still other couples use the vibrator as part of sex play to help the woman achieve orgasm. Some couples use vibrator stimulation during intercourse to increase clitoral stimulation, which allows the woman to be orgasmic during coitus. The vibrator is not just the woman's device; many men enjoy giving and receiving vibrator stimulation.

Some uses of the vibrator might appeal to you; others might strike you as strange or "kinky." Our message is not that you have to try it, but that this is one more option to consider as a way to enhance sexual pleasure.

ANAL STIMULATION

Typically, people associate the anus with dirtiness. What people do not realize is that the anal area contains a large number of nerve endings. The anal area is an erogenous zone just as is the mons and labia or the shaft of the penis and testicles. Some people express a good deal of interest in and arousal from having their buttocks touched and stroked. Many couples enjoy rear-entry penis-vagina intercourse because of contact with the buttocks. Both men and women can enjoy manual stimulation around the perineum and anal area. Many couples engage in buttock and anal stimulation and find it pleasurable.

When people think of anal sex, they are specifically referring to anal intercourse. About one in four couples had experimented with anal intercourse until the recent concern over AIDS. Anal intercourse, especially the passive role, is the most dangerous technique for the transmission of the HIV virus. We strongly urge couples to refrain from anal intercourse unless they are sure both are HIV negative.

There are many myths about this sexual practice, the most prominent being that it is a sign of "latent homosexuality." That term is probably the most misused of any in sexual language. The concept of latent homosexuality is used as a club to keep couples from experimenting sexually because of a fear that they will unleash latent, perverse tendencies. There is no such thing as an exclusive homosexual behavior. Gay couples interact sexually in basically the same way as do heterosexual couples. What makes sex homosexual is that it is engaged in by two people of the *same* sex, not the sexual behavior itself.

Anal intercourse is prepared for by using a lubricant to facilitate entry. Since the anal sphincter muscle does not easily dilate, entry should be slow and guided by the woman so she does not experience pain. Many couples report discomfort on the first few insertions, but as they communicate and develop a comfortable style of insertion the problem dissipates. One of the advantages of anal intercourse is that the male can simultaneously provide hand stimulation of the vulva and clitoral area. Many couples enjoy the sensations of anal as opposed to vaginal intercourse. A major warning is not to switch from anal to vaginal intercourse because bacteria from the anus can infect the vagina. He can use a lubricated condom during anal intercourse and remove it for vaginal intercourse. Or he could wash his penis before engaging in vaginal intercourse. This same guidance applies to manual stimulation inside the anus; wash your hands before doing vaginal stimulation.

Many couples find manual stimulation around the buttocks and anal area more pleasurable than actual insertion. It has all the advantages of stimulating the nerve endings and providing different sensations with none of the disadvantages of insertion. Manual anal stimulation is usually done in the context of other sexual activity, such as intercourse, or breast or penile stimulation. Anal stimulation can be pleasurable activity to add to the totality of your sexual encounter.

USE OF SEXUALLY EXPLICIT MATERIALS (EROTICA)

What is the difference between R-rated and X-rated movies? It is the difference between a romantic and sensual yet explicit view of sex and a nonromantic but graphic and sometimes violent or degrading presentation of the sexual encounter. Whether presented in a motion picture, magazine photographs, or a novel, the purpose is to break down inhibitions and excite you by providing the details of sexual scenarios. Like fantasies, the erotic experiences depicted might not be what you want to do, but watching or reading about them can arouse you.

Sharing sexually explicit material can be a couple activity, instead of a man going alone to a stag party and/or sneaking magazines to the office to read. Many couples become excited by watching a video or looking at pictures and sharing their arousal. Feelings of shared illicitness add to arousal. Erotica, or sexually explicit material, can be arousing for both women and men. The VCR has revolutionized the use of erotic videotapes. Previously, people had to go to distinctly unsavory X-rated movie houses. Erotica, X-rated videos, novels, magazines, or pictures can be shared in the privacy of your home.

A problem with pornographic materials is that they most often present an aggressive, male-dominant, performance-oriented, and degrading view of sexuality. The men always have super-large erections and can have orgasm after orgasm. The women always have big breasts and appear to enjoy the painful and acrobatic aspects of the encounter. Sex is impersonal but always perfectly performed. The message is "the best sex is dirty sex." Isn't this opposed to what we've written concerning intimacy, warmth, and nondemand pleasuring? Of course, and yet isn't there also something exciting about occasionally having a quick "fuck" or fantasizing a passionate sexual encounter with a stranger? Looking at or reading erotica is a way to experience vicariously a wide variety of sexually stimulating situations without feeling guilty or pressured to play them out. Choose erotica that can be arousing for both partners. Avoid erotica that displeases or intimidates either partner.

GROUP SEX

Radical sexual theorists believe the eptiome of sexual libera-
tion is the experience of group ambisexuality (the ability to
engage in same sex, opposite sex, and solo sex activity in a
group setting). We believe this emphasis on finding the ultimate
sexual behavior to prove you're liberated is a new form of
sexual fascism.

Group sex is a sexual variant some couples might choose to
experiment with. It has the potential to be sexually exciting, but
can be destructive to the couple's bond. Experimenting with
group sex should be undertaken only if you have carefully
discussed your feelings and motivations as well as agreed on a
plan to bail out of the experiment if it becomes uncomfortable
or destructive. In this age of sexually transmitted diseases and
AIDS, it is crucial that you know the health status of other
people you engage with sexually, and that you utilize safe sex
techniques.

There are many varieties of group sex, including organized
swinging (either open to observation by others or done pri-
vately), bisexual group encounters, simultaneous group sex fea-
turing "daisy chains," and the use of threesomes. The major
enticement is to give and receive varying kinds of sexual stimulation with a variety of partners. The experience of fellating
someone and at the same time having intercourse, of three
people stimulating you simultaneously, or of having vaginal and
anal intercourse at the same time can provide a great deal of
sexual excitement. Another source of arousal is observing people engaging in a variety of sexual interactions. Some men
report feeling very excited watching their wife and another
woman engaging in cunnilingus, or a woman may become
aroused when watching two women stimulating her husband.
This illustrates the major psychological drawback of group sex:
fears of jealousy, performance comparisons, and a sense of
alienating, impersonal sex. The major health concern is exposure to multiple partners with the ensuing danger of sexually
transmitted diseases.

Advocates of group sex claim it is a sharing of multiple
pleasures in which openness and honesty overcome jealousy and

the relationships are caring and nonmanipulative. Those who disparage group sex, including some who had previously engaged in it, see it as more attractive in theory than in practice. Couples rationalize bad feelings, but eventually one or both people feel manipulated, used, jealous, and/or distrustful. The empirical data indicates that group sex is destructive to most couples' marital and sexual relationship. We do not advise group sexual experimentation. For those who do engage in group sex it is imperative that they protect their health and utilize safe sex techniques.

CLOSING THOUGHTS

In summarizing this chapter, our theme is that there are a range of sexual variations and techniques that could provide excitement to revitalize your sexual relationship. We have discussed several alternatives, some of which we've incorporated into our lives and others we have chosen not to use, either because they don't interest us or we feel they would harm our relationship. You can decide which, if any, of these scenarios and techniques would be pleasurable and enhancing for you as a couple.

The essence of creative sexuality does not lie in techniques. The most genuine and satisfying components of marital sex are an awareness of your feelings and desires and comfort in communicating these to your spouse. Sex is most creative not when it focuses on isolated techniques, but when it involves you as a person being intimately aware of yourself and your spouse, sharing yourselves as a sexual couple.

8
CONCEPTION, CONTRACEPTION, AND INFERTILITY

One of the most emotionally complex and important decisions a couple make is whether or not to have children. Traditionally, the main function of sex was procreation. To be married without children was socially deviant.

In the last generation, with the emphasis on planned, wanted children, conception has shifted from a cultural "should" to a choice, especially in terms of the number of children. Sexuality is viewed more broadly as shared pleasure, a means to reinforce and deepen intimacy, and as a tension reducer. Conception is a potential function of sexuality, not its main function. Children are not necessary to justify sexuality or a marriage. Ideally, a child would be planned and wanted, an affirmation of the couple bond and desire to be a family.

The issues of conception, contraception, and infertility are difficult and complex. The United States has the highest premarital pregnancy rate of any Western country. Approximately one in three women has an unplanned premarital pregnancy. Approximately one in four brides is pregnant at the time of marriage and for teenage brides it is over 70 percent. Three-quarters of all couples find it all too easy to get pregnant; their concern is using contraception to prevent unwanted pregnancies. One out of four couples experiences difficulty becoming pregnant, and more than 10 percent are infertile.

We will present guidelines for increasing awareness and decision-making in this complex area of conception, contraception, and family planning. There is no one right answer for all couples. The decision to have children is individual and value-laden. The traditional view was that the right choice was to have children, with the implication that to decide otherwise was an indication of immaturity, selfishness, or hostility to traditional values. Couples need to examine their attitudes, feelings, values, and life situations, and determine what is in their best interests. A child is at least an eighteen-year commitment—financially, practically, and most of all emotionally. Pregnancy and child rearing is a choice, not a mandate. Whether to have a child is one of the most important decisions a couple makes, and one of the most difficult to reverse. People—especially mothers—can switch careers, marriages, and living arrangements more easily than they can cease parenting.

There are few decisions in life that are as emotionally complex as whether to have children, when to have them, and how many to have. We have counseled competent, successful couples who have no trouble making million-dollar professional decisions, but absolutely wilt under the stress of a family planning choice. Choosing to have a child is fundamentally an emotional decision. If couples decided only on the basis of financial, practical, and logical factors, no one would choose to have a child and the human race would disappear. Just the opposite is happening—this planet is faced with a population explosion, especially in developing countries, that threatens the earth's resources. Population planning is one of the most important issues facing the world community.

The primary emotional reasons that couples choose to have children is to experience the process of pregnancy, and to participate in parenting a baby and watching her grow into an independent person. Pregnancy, childbirth, and parenting are among life's unique and special experiences, and most couples do choose to have children. Those individuals and couples who decide the opposite deserve to have their choice respected and supported. If couples carefully considered the decision, up to 30 percent might choose to remain childless. The time, as well as the financial and emotional commitment children require is truly daunting. Nevertheless the decision to be childless should be made not out of fear, but as a positive commitment to individual growth and to the life of the couple. Couples without children report high levels of emotional and sexual satisfaction.

WAIT UNTIL MID-TWENTIES FOR MARRIAGE AND CHILDREN

Our principal guideline is that a couple should delay the time they marry—perferably to their early or mid-twenties—and wait at least two years in order to strengthen their marital bond before becoming pregnant. Although this concept is becoming more accepted, the majority of couples do not follow it. The average age to marry is twenty-five for males and twenty-three for females, but the modal (single most frequent) age to marry is eighteen for women and twenty for men. Approximately one in four brides is pregnant at the time of marriage, and the typical couple have their first child within eighteen months of marriage. By age thirty most people are married and have a child, and many have two or more children.

Empirical research indicates that individuals would be wise to establish their own autonomy and complete vocational or career training before making the commitment to marriage. Marrying between twenty-three and twenty-seven and beginning child-bearing at twenty-five to thirty allows for the establishment of a stronger base for the marital relationship as well as family and parenting roles. This conceptualization, like other guidelines and viewpoints expressed throughout the book, is based on both research and clinical data. There are tremendous individual differences among couples in experience, values, attitudes, and maturity. This determines whether a guideline is viable for a specific couple. These guidelines provide information and a framework for you to discuss and utilize for decision-making. We were married when Barry was twenty-three and Emily twenty-one, and had our first child two years and one month later, barely within the guideline.

One of the first tasks in marriage is to establish norms and expectations that facilitate the development of intimacy and security. It's important that each person maintain his own individuality; being a couple does not negate individual interests and values.

Bob and Susan. They married when Bob was twenty-five and Susan twenty-four, after knowing each other two years and living together six months. Both were starting in their chosen careers. Although they'd discussed what they wanted from marriage, as with most couples it was not until they were actually married and dealing with everyday realities that their idealized and intellectualized concepts of marriage were made immediate. Intimacy was something they had talked extensively about when living together, but once married they discovered an added dimension. Susan was wary of becoming overly dependent on Bob, yet both wanted trust, intimacy, and security in their marriage. Each, in effect, was asking, "How can I be my own person yet still be a loving and intimate spouse?" They wanted to maintain individual interests and friends as well as cultivate couple activities and friends.

In the first year of marriage they experienced more conflict than during the previous year. In the heat of an argument Bob would say that they just should have continued living together. Hearing this, Susan became both angry and anxious. She felt angry at Bob for his disparagement and lack of commitment, and anxious because she felt her security threatened. Bob's outburst was his way of asserting the traditional masculine role and distancing himself from Susan. Like most males, he thought that he needed intimacy and security less than a woman. Yet when he was honest, Bob knew he had married not for practical and societal reasons but out of a genuine desire to be with Susan and to meet his needs for security and intimacy. He wanted a marriage in which he could be himself and safely communicate his doubts and vulnerabilities as well as his strengths and hopes.

After unsettling arguments, they would discuss whether having a child might bring greater stability and provide a stronger family atmosphere. Susan had taken a college course on the changing roles of women, and knew that for women in their twenties it was extremely difficult to manage a marriage, career, and children simultaneously. It was either the career or the marriage that broke down. Although planned, wanted children are beneficial to a couple's relationship, the birth of a first child is a major transition and puts stress on a marital bond. Susan and Bob wisely decided to postpone consideration of children for another year and, instead, to focus their energy on building a stronger and more cohesive marital bond. They communicated and supported one another, but had a difficult time arguing constructively. They were not enjoying social activities or couple time as much as they would have liked, and their sex life was becoming "the same old thing." In other words, they were starting to fall into the traps that lurk in marriage. They desired a satisfying marital life, but did not put energy into making it happen and had allowed things to slide toward mediocrity.

Susan resented being responsible for birth control. Early in the relationship Bob used condoms, but neither particularly liked them. Susan had tried an IUD (intrauterine device, see p. 63), but disliked the resultant cramping and heavy bleeding. She preferred a diaphragm to the IUD, but did not like having to insert it each time they had sex and having to keep it in six hours after his ejaculation. It was their discouragement with other forms of birth control that led them eventually to the birth control pill. Susan had no problems with the pill, but it seemed unfair that the burden for birth control was on her shoulders.

Sex is naturally exciting during the first weeks and months of a new relationship. Even though Bob ejaculated early and Susan had difficulty reaching orgasm, theirs was arousing sex. After eight months, Bob attained good ejaculatory control and Susan was regularly orgasmic. This was accomplished by openly talking about sexuality and experimenting with sexual scenarios and techniques, especially using slower coital thrusting and Susan showing Bob how to use two fingers to stimulate her clitoral area. Even more important, there was a sense of caring and a feeling of working together.

Once the sexual relationship was functional, there was a decrease in communication and experimentation. They fell into the trap of believing that once they could do it well, there was nothing left to learn and no reason to experiment further. Sexuality stagnates when no new energy is expended. After six months, Bob was finding sex routine and mechanical. Susan did not have sexual daydreams about Bob anymore, romance had disappeared, and she had to work at being orgasmic rather than its being a naturally flowing response. In trying to ascertain why the pleasure had gone out of their sex and what to do about it, they considered several alternatives, including sex therapy, techniques from sex manuals, and extramarital affairs. They read articles in popular magazines and found themselves confused by the dogmatic and often contradictory advice. Bob and Susan were having a hard time facing up to their sexual problem; they had allowed the sense of creative and intimate sex to dissipate. They were no longer sharing experiences, interacting in a caring manner, being spontaneous, aware of each other's moods, and matching sexual interaction to their feelings. When they were a loving and intimate couple—more affectionate and playful *outside* the bedroom, and more sensuous and spontaneous during sex itself—there was a sexual reawakening. They put pleasure back into their sexuality.

The issues faced by Susan and Bob will occur not only in the first year or two but throughout the entire marriage. Pleasure and sexual functioning are not resolved once and for all, but continue to arise during the marriage. Even if you find sex very satisfying at twenty-five, you will face new sexual issues at thirty-five, forty-five, fifty-five, sixty-five, and seventy-five— in fact, as long as you are a sexual couple. This is not a sign of a poor marriage; it is a healthy sign. You are changing as people and your marital relationship is changing, so of course your sexual relationship not only can change but should. This is equally true of your communication process, enjoyment of each other, and constructive argument.

At this point, Bob and Susan were ready to discuss children. They knew couples who had decided not to have children. Couples need to consider carefully whether their desire to have children is based on what is expected, or on whether their parents want grandchildren. In the best of all worlds, a couple would not have children unless they were reasonably sure they had a stable marriage and were willing to make an eighteen-year commitment to parenting. Some couples would be better off in their life and marriage if they decided not to parent.

After discussing the emotional, financial, psychological, and practical pros and cons, Susan and Bob chose to have children. They were pleased that they'd waited two and a half years before trying to get pregnant. They needed that time to solidify their marital and sexual bond. Susan stopped taking birth control pills, and they were happy to be among those couples who find becoming pregnant fun and easy. It was great having intercourse without worry about contraception. There is something very special about wondering if this is the time you will conceive. Trying to become pregnant is a major stimulus to sexual desire and the most natural aphrodisiac.

Steve and Judy. In many ways, Steve and Judy were a typical couple, marrying when Steve was twenty-three and Judy twenty-one. They decided to postpone children while Steve completed his graduate work. Since there were few financial responsibilities, Judy decided to obtain further career training. Five years later, both were involved in their careers, doing well financially, and they had the money and time for a three-week vacation and skiing weekends. Both, but especially Judy, began getting parental pressure to start a family. There were subtle hints that they were becoming too selfish and that if they waited much longer, it would be difficult for them to adjust to the stresses and demands of children. Many of their friends were settling down, buying homes, and having babies. They were beginning to feel like social outcasts who were not keeping up with the Joneses. What Steve and Judy experienced were the subtle and not so subtle cultural expectations and pressures to have a family. Actually, Steve was more interested in having children than Judy. She enjoyed her career, their couple freedom, and flexible lifestyle, and felt little inclination to become pregnant. They had to defend and justify their choice to themselves, their families, and friends. They felt—and rightly so— that this was a legitimate decision for them, and Steve had a vasectomy at thirty-one.

MYTHS IN FAMILY PLANNING

In considering the issue of children, there is no all-purpose, right decision. Be aware of popular myths about children:

1. The more the merrier.
2. An only child is usually maladjusted.
3. You must have your first child by thirty.
4. Under no circumstances should you have children after forty.
5. It is crucial to have both boys and girls.
6. Planning children takes the love and spontaneity out of sex.
7. Having children stabilizes a rocky marriage.

We suggest the following guidelines for family planning:

1. Having children should be a choice agreed to by both partners.
2. Ideally, the couple relationship would be on a solid footing emotionally, sexually, and financially before the choice to have a child.
3. A couple should wait at least two years before beginning a family.
4. Children should be planned and wanted.
5. Children are at least an eighteen-year commitment. Parents should consider their financial resources and psychological readiness to make this commitment.

CONTRACEPTION AND STERILIZATION

There is no perfect contraceptive. A perfect contraceptive would have the following characteristics: (1) be totally effective, (2) have no immediate or long-term side effects, (3) be separate from sexual activity, (4) be easily reversible, (5) require little or no effort on the part of the user, (6) could be used by male or female, (7) be inexpensive. Nothing presently available comes close to meeting these criteria. A couple can choose the pill, diaphragm, IUD, or condoms. There are other, less effective forms of birth control—foam, jelly, rhythm, cervical sponge—but the first four are the best.

The birth control pill is the most effective form of contraception presently available. It must be taken daily and functions by preventing ovulation. Lower levels of estrogen have made the pill safer, with reduced side effects. It is important to choose a gynecologist who is knowledgeable about current research and different brands of birth control pills. It is crucial that the gynecologist knows your full medical history and monitors your health on a yearly basis. Women who have a family history of blood clotting or stroke are not good candidates for the pill, nor are older women who smoke. A major advantage of the pill is that it separates the contraceptive act from the sexual act. But a woman has to maintain motivation to take the pill each day. If one is forgotten or missed, take it as soon as possible. If more than twelve hours have elapsed, the usual advice is to utilize a back-up contraceptive for the rest of the cycle.

The diaphragm is one of the oldest forms of birth control. It has two major advantages: it is highly effective when used properly and has virtually no medical side effects. A gynecologist must properly fit the diaphragm, which is a rubber-based ring inserted inside the vagina. The diaphragm blocks conception in two ways. The device itself serves as a barrier covering the cervix so that sperm cannot penetrate. Just as vital, a spermicidal jelly is placed around and inside it and serves to kill sperm. The spermicide needs to be placed on the diaphragm no sooner than two hours, and preferably closer to an hour, before beginning intercourse. The diaphragm must be left in place at least six hours after intercourse. If you desire to have intercourse a second time, you must use a special inserter to apply another dose of spermicidal jelly while the diaphragm remains in place. The key to successful use is the commitment to use it on every sexual occasion no matter how aroused you are.

Condoms are experiencing a revived popularity because they are the only contraceptive that also protects against sexually transmitted diseases such as AIDS. They are also the only male contraceptive, and couples who value shared responsibility sometimes employ the condom in conjunction with the diaphragm or foam. Some couples begin intercourse and, as arousal builds, withdraw and put on a condom, which is unsafe. Proper use of condoms includes putting the condom on before insertion, leaving a small space at the end to catch the semen, and being sure that the male withdraws soon after ejaculation and holds the condom at the base of the penis so it doesn't slip off. Although condoms are safe, readily accessible, and good contraceptives, they are not as effective as the pill, diaphragm, or IUD.

The IUD is one of the most controversial contraceptives because one type, the Dalkon Shield, was defective and resulted in serious injury to many women. Newer and safer IUD models have been introduced. It is crucial to consult a gynecologist who is current on IUD research and skilled at insertion. No one knows precisely how the IUD works, but it appears to interfere with the implantation of the ovum in the uterus. Those who are successful with the IUD say they have effective contraception without worrying about taking a pill each day or inserting a diaphragm before each intercourse. However, because of concerns about its safety, and the heavy menstrual bleeding it sometimes causes, the IUD is no longer a widely used contraceptive.

The reason sterilization is the most popular form of birth control for couples over thirty is that they've become frustrated with and discouraged by contraception. Yet, if you want to avoid an unwanted pregnancy, the answer is a couple commitment to regular use of contraception. Approximately 40 percent of marital pregnancies are unplanned, although that does not mean the baby is unwanted.

The decision to undergo sterilization should not be made lightly. Although microsurgery has made it easier to reverse a vasectomy, both vasectomy and tubal ligation are best thought of as permanent methods. Whether a man should get a vasectomy or a woman have a tubal ligation is difficult and subjective decision. If the couple are sure they do not want additional children, they need to discuss carefully the range of factors—medical, psychological, sexual, and motivational—to determine who should undertake surgery. The spouse who is more committed to not having additional children, less vulnerable to psychological or sexual worries, and more confident about surgery is the one who should volunteer. From a strictly medical viewpoint, the vasectomy is the simpler, safer, and less costly procedure. Paradoxically, about three times more women have tubal ligations than males who choose vasectomies. This is a side effect of the double standard in which conception, contraception, and children are viewed as the responsibility of women.

ENJOYING PREGNANCY AS A COUPLE

Since it takes two to conceive a child, there is every reason to join together during the pregnancy, in prepared-childbirth classes, in the delivery room, and parenting the baby. The traditional view is that childbirth and babies are strictly the concern of women, and that men have only minimal interest and involvement. It is no wonder that the most typical time for a couple to separate or for a man to begin an extramarital affair is three months before or three months after the birth of a first child. He feels left out of her life and the pregnancy experience, and has no sexual outlet. Let us look at a couple where the problems were anticipated and handled with a more satisfying outcome.

Jack and Roberta. In the heat of passion, Jack and Roberta had forgotten to use a diaphragm, and Roberta became pregnant. After a great deal of discussion, they decided that, although this pregnancy was not planned, they did want the child. Further, Roberta had a strong desire—and with some prodding, Jack agreed—to be actively involved in the preparation and actual childbirth procedure. They chose an obstetrician who was enthusiastic about prepared childbirth and who would allow Jack to be present in the labor and delivery room. They enjoyed taking the prepared childbirth course, practicing the exercises at home, and discussing the transitions a new baby would bring to their lives. Roberta and Jack communicated their sexual feelings and needs. They found, as do many couples, that Roberta was sexually responsive during the second trimester of her pregnancy (due to an increase in pelvic vasocongestion in the woman as well as—possibly—relief over no longer having morning sickness). Roberta was thrilled to be multiorgasmic for the first time in her life.

As she became larger and felt more awkward in her last trimester, they discussed alternative intercourse positions and nonintercourse sexual outlets. Their favorite late-stage intercourse position was Roberta sitting on the sofa with a pillow supporting her back with her vulva at the edge of the sofa. Jack knelt on three cushions, both for comfort and to raise himself so that his penis was directly in front of her vagina. There was no pressure on Roberta's stomach, which is the crucial factor during the late stages of pregnancy. Jack could fondle her breasts, mons, and clitoral area and Roberta could massage Jack's testicles and inner thighs during coitus. They liked this position so well that they continued using it after the pregnancy. They also used side-by-side intercourse positions and especially liked a rear-entry position in which Roberta was half on her side so there was minimal pressure on her stomach. There were times when Jack wanted sexual release, but Roberta felt that intercourse would be uncomfortable. She would manually or orally stimulate him to orgasm. At other times, he would masturbate. Roberta made it clear that even when she felt heavy, awkward, and not sexual, she still desired affectionate touching. She liked being stroked and held and took pleasure from sexually satisfying Jack. Roberta and Jack valued the closeness they shared during the pregnancy.

The birth itself was one of the peak experiences in Jack and Roberta's lives. Although there was discomfort and pain, the classes and exercises paid off. Roberta experienced a great deal of fulfillment in being awake and alert at the birth of her daughter. Jack's active involvement and presence was more gratifying to him than he'd anticipated, and much more fulfilling than the role of an inept father pacing in the waiting room. Roberta remained in the hospital three days, and they had "rooming in." This allowed them to become accustomed to the tasks of parenthood—changing diapers, giving feedings, and gaining confidence being with the baby.

One of the major issues in the transition to being a family is not to lose track of your husband-wife bond. This is especially true of the sexual relationship. Motherhood does not mean the woman becomes less sexual. Couples need to devote time to reestablishing their sexual relationship while being aware of the stresses and strains of parenting a baby. This can be a hard time for a couple; it certainly was for us (our first child was a non-sleeper). Lack of sleep can inhibit sexual desire. Put the time and energy into coping with this transition so you look back on the experience as one that has strengthened your bond rather than subverted it.

Having children is a choice. It is our prediction that in the future more couples will choose not to have children. Freedom from the responsibility of parenting allows greater degrees of freedom in a couple's lifestyle, career plans, financial status, and ability to travel. Children are great financial as well as psychological responsibilities, especially if these responsibilities are viewed as a burden instead of a choice. The primary reason to have children is a genuine desire and commitment to the growth and development of another human being. Choosing to have children involves making a commitment to share yourself emotionally, physically, financially, and psychologically for an eighteen-year period.

INFERTILITY

Approximately 25 percent of couples have difficulty conceiving. Infertility problems put inordinate stress on the couple bond, partly because they are so unexpected. Most people assume they will have no trouble becoming pregnant. It is extremely upsetting and frustrating to discover that what is so easy for so many couples is difficult and could prove impossible for you. If you are one out of four couples facing infertility problems, the first guideline is not to blame yourself or question your masculinity or femininity.

There are a host of causes for fertility problems. Those that affect women include failure to ovulate, blocked fallopian tubes, an incompetent cervix, high vaginal acidity, endometriosis, and vaginismus. About 40 percent of fertility problems involve male disorders, which include low sperm counts, erection problems, poor sperm motility, and ejaculatory inhibition. A fertility problem is best viewed as a couple problem and not as a cause for blame or guilt. It puts enormous stress on the person's sense of well-being, on the couple bond, and on the sexual relationship. If a couple has not been able to conceive after twelve months of trying, we suggest a referral to an infertility specialist. If the problem is not resolved in six months, we suggest consulting a marital therapist and/or an infertility support group to help you deal with the psychological, relational, and sexual stress caused by fertility problems.

A specific problem is isolated and easily treated in about 25 percent of couples. The remainder have to deal with a number of medical techniques including drugs to promote ovulation, microsurgery to open the fallopian tubes, varicocele surgery, or hormone treatment to improve sperm functioning. Couples engage in sex therapy to deal with vaginismus, erection problems, or ejaculatory inhibition. Artificial insemination with either the husband's or a donor's sperm has been successful for many couples. There are a number of new, expensive, and difficult technological breakthroughs such as *in vitro* fertilization. Unless one has experienced it, it's hard to imagine the individual and couple stress caused by a fertility problem.

Margaret and Frank. When Margaret was sixteen she had an unplanned pregnancy. After talking with her parents and consulting her minister, Margaret decided to continue the pregnancy and give the baby up for adoption. Although this was a distressing experience for her, she planned to become pregnant and have a child after she was married. She was proud to have graduated high school with her class and expected to marry after completing college. Margaret entered her twenties as Americans were undergoing a dramatic change in patterns of dating and marrying. She did not marry Frank (he was thirty-two and this was his second marriage) until she was twenty-eight. Frank wanted to wait at least three years before beginning a family. When they began having intercourse without contraception, Margaret was enthusiastic and optimistic. Her enthusiasm turned to frustration and then panic when they did not become pregnant within a year. Margaret was thirty-two and terrified that she would not be able to have children.

The infertility specialist they consulted was technically expert, but not particularly empathic or forthcoming with information (a typical complaint about infertility specialists). Margaret and Frank chose to stay with him because of his excellent professional reputation, but decided to consult a marriage therapist to deal with emotional stress, help them discuss alternatives, and to problem solve. Medical assessment indicated that Frank's sperm were impaired in terms of motility; there was blockage in Margaret's fallopian tubes, and the post-coital test indicated that Frank's sperm were not progressing through the cervix in sufficient numbers. As the months rolled by, Frank felt sexual pressure which resulted in erection problems during the high-probability week. Margaret found that sex on a timetable lowered her sexual desire. The marriage therapist suggested that Margaret and Frank emphasize pleasurable, spontaneous sex during the rest of the month. They needed that time to reenergize their marital and sexual bond. This was a helpful suggestion, but the reality was that the task-oriented sex of the high-probability week was no fun.

It was the marital therapist who suggested that they try insemination with Frank's sperm. The infertility specialist thought this was a good idea, because from the viewpoint of efficacy insemination is a more successful way of becoming pregnant than intercourse. Frank and Margaret were initially ambivalent—Frank because he saw it as a sign of failure, and Margaret because it seemed too clinical. However, as they discussed their feelings and perceptions, they became more comfortable with the idea. They were scheduled to do two inseminations during the high-probability week, and were encouraged to have intercourse after the second insemination. They were not sure whether the resulting pregnancy came from insemination or intercourse, and they frankly didn't care.

Anita and Jonathan. Jonathan was an accountant and a very precise fellow. He didn't like leaving things to chance, so when they tried to get pregnant he insisted they employ fertility enhancement procedures. They used an over-the-counter device to determine when Anita ovulated. They had intercourse the day before she was to ovulate and the day she ovulated. Jonathan had read that it was important to have intercourse in the man-on-top position, that he thrust deeply before ejaculation and withdraw immediately after he ejaculated, and that she stay in that position with her knees bent for twenty minutes to facilitate the sperm swimming through the cervix. They followed this format rigorously for six months and when they did not become pregnant Jonathan insisted that they consult an infertility specialist. He willingly gave a sperm sample with the full expectation that it would be fine. He was anxious to go ahead with testing of Anita to pinpoint the problem, and was shocked to discover that he produced very few sperm and the prognosis was negative that he could cause conception. He consulted two urologists with a subspecialty in infertility who confirmed the diagnosis. Jonathan was used to feeling in control of his life, his profession, and his ability to make numbers come out right. He was dismayed that he couldn't do this in an area that seemed as easy and natural as conception.

Anita's personal strength helped them through this crisis. She made it clear that she valued Jonathan as a spouse, lover, and person. There is no connection between fertility and masculinity or sexual prowess. Anita had always valued their sex life, and had found the pregnancy enhancement procedures off-putting.

She initiated sexual play more during the month following the information about his sperm count than at any time in the marriage. Jonathan was a reluctant sex partner, but as Anita emphasized the importance and quality of their sexual relationship, Jonathan gradually emerged from his depression and became a fully involved intimate partner.

Anita took the lead in discussing alternative means to parent a child. They considered adopting a hard-to-place child, using insemination with donor sperm, adopting a foreign infant, trying surrogate parenting, and having foster children. Although these alternatives might work for other couples, Jonathan and Anita opted to proceed with adoption through their local Catholic Charities agency. Jonathan joked that between writing an autobiography, going through a detailed personal and family history, having a social worker visit and assess their home, and getting letters of reference, adopting a child was a much more rigorous procedure than biologically having a baby. The adoption process certainly causes the couple to carefully consider their motivation to parent. If couples had to do this before becoming pregnant, our estimate is that at least a quarter would opt to remain childless. Anita and Jonathan maintained their motivation and "jumped through the hoops." The process took over two years, but they adopted a six-month-old girl and two years later a one-month-old boy.

CLOSING THOUGHTS

Conception, contraception, and infertility are among the most complex and value-laden issues a couple faces. Discussing attitudes, values, and feelings, and reaching decisions both people can live with is vital. One of the most important decisions a couple makes is whether to have children, and, if yes, when and how many. The process involves the attitudes, plans, and, most important, the emotional commitment of both people. We are strongly in favor of planned, wanted children. Although that's the ideal, it is the exception rather than the rule.

No matter what decision you make, remember you are a couple first. The most important relationship in a family is the husband-wife bond. If you keep it strong and viable, parenting will go better for you as well as your children.

9

PARENTS AS SEX EDUCATORS

Children are sexual from the day they're born. Within a few hours, even minutes, of birth, females vaginally lubricate and males have an erection. Children are aware of their bodies and of male-female genital differences at a very young age. They have sexual feelings and responses throughout childhood that greatly increase during adolescence. Parents who ignore sexual realities face a crisis as their children become adolescents and young adults.

The conflicts adolescent children experience often confuse or exacerbate sexual concerns of parents. Behind most views about children's sexuality is *fear*—fear that the adolescent will contract a sexually transmitted disease, become pregnant, be sexually abused, or be emotionally damaged in a destructive relationship. Parents sometimes hope to delay the onset of sexual feelings and conflicts by ignoring their children's sexuality, a useless and self-defeating strategy. Parents who do not have a good marital sexual relationship or had harmful sexual experiences in childhood or adolescent years find this aspect of child development particularly conflictual, bringing forth feelings of personal and parental inadequacy.

To eliminate this cycle of fear and conflict, the first priority for parents is to develop an understanding of, and comfort with, their own sexuality. Those who provide a positive model of knowledge and comfort establish an excellent base for family sex education. Perhaps the best sex education for a child is to see Mom and Dad kissing in the kitchen or being affectionate in the family room. Parents who verbally and behaviorally give a clear message that affection, sexuality, and love are good provide a solid basis for the child's view of relationships and sexuality.

Parents who are aware that they are not only mother and father, but also husband and wife, are better able to deal with family sexuality issues. The basis of family sexuality is the comfortable and positive sexual bond between husband and wife.

Marge and John. Marge and John had been married twenty-seven years. For the past eight they'd had sexual difficulties because of John's intermittent erectile problems. During the most recent two years John had been unable to have intercourse, which finally caused them to seek sex therapy. Partly because of discomfort over this sexual problem, the children's sex education was "education by omission." There were few sex talks between mother and daughter or father and son. Parental sex education consisted of vague warnings to "stay out of trouble." In retrospect, Marge and John regretted not being positive sex educators nor askable parents. At the time of treatment, their son was twenty-five and their daughter twenty-one, and both were unmarried.

Sex therapy was successful because John and Marge cared about each other and were open to learning new communication and sexual techniques. Like many couples with sexual difficulties, the combination of performance anxiety and misunderstanding resulted in a self-perpetuating cycle of fearful anticipation, bad sexual experiences, and then prolonged sexual avoidance. The outcome was a decrease in communication and affection. Replacing this self-defeating pattern with an openness to nondemand touching, pleasure-orientation, and multiple stimulation, they gradually regained comfort and confidence with erections, allowing sex once again to be a satisfying part of their marital bond. Often it is not loss of ability to function, but loss of comfort and confidence that causes erectile problems.

This newfound comfort extended to telling their young adult children that they were seeing a therapist to improve their marital and sexual relationship. Parental sharing of this information had noticeable positive effects. The adult children shared their concerns about relationships, and their fears that Marge and John were disappointed because of their premarital sexual activity. John and Marge assured their adult children that they loved them, cared about them, and did not want to judge them. They did reaffirm their belief that sex reached its ultimate satisfaction in an intimate, committed marital relationship. The entire family would have benefitted if John and Marge had attended to their sexual relationship earlier. Such attention not only would have helped them as husband and wife, but would have provided the whole family with a more open and comfortable basis for discussing sexual feelings and values, and would have helped them to become positive sex educators for their children.

FAMILY SEXUALITY ISSUES

Even when adults are not doing well sexually—if they have divorced, or the couple do not feel close sexually, or one parent continues to feel victimized by a childhood sexual trauma, or there has been an extramarital affair or a sexual dysfunction recently—parents can still provide positive information, attitudes, and values to their children. Although such information has more impact if the parents are a good model for sexual attitudes and functioning, parents—like other adults—may be sexually dysfunctional or be dealing with difficult relationship issues. Being a parent does not mean you pretend to be perfect and have all the answers.

Family sexuality education is a continually occurring process. The child's sex education begins at the moment of birth. Sex is a lifelong, natural physiological function, like breathing. Not only the mother but both parents touching and holding the baby

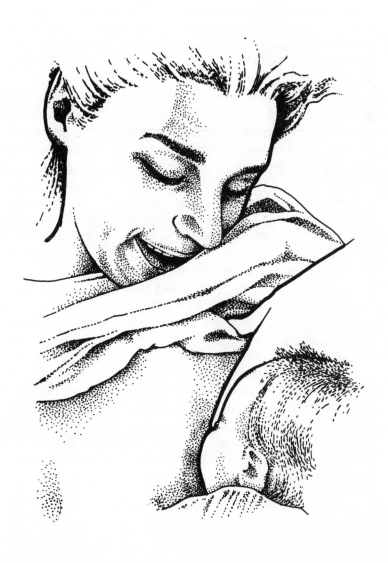

Breast-feeding helps the mother-child bonding process and can be very fulfilling for the woman.

provide contact comfort and crucial learning about caring, trust, and security. Feeling good about one's body and enjoyment of touching forms the basis of sexual functioning, and begins early in life. This is equally true for male and female babies. In our culture, male babies receive less holding and cuddling. We encourage father and mother to hold and touch male and female children.

Before the child is a year, she will begin exploring her genitals, a natural aspect of body awareness. Since there are more nerve endings in the genital region than any other part of the body, the child experiences pleasure from genital touching and will continue. Instead of the parent becoming anxious, slapping the child's hands, and saying "no"—certainly a negative message about her body and genitals—the parent can accept body exploration as natural and healthy. The child should learn proper words for genitals: penis and vulva rather than "ding-dong," "down there," or "whatsit." Formerly, a girl was told she was different from her brother because she did not have a penis. It is better to say, "You are a girl and you have a vulva, your brother is a boy and he has a penis."

As children develop, especially in the four to six age range, issues regarding privacy, nudity, and genital touching come to the forefront. The parental message should continue to be positive. The child can be comfortable with his body, genitals, and nudity, but should learn that there are appropriate and inappropriate contexts. This is important and valuable knowledge. Your sexuality is a good part of you as a person, but you have to learn appropriate times and situations to express it. Specific guidelines can be individualized and governed by the parents' value system and comfort level.

Judy and Bob. Judy and Bob were raised in homes where nudity was not allowed and displays of physical affection were restricted to special events, such as birthdays, and consisted simply of a hug and kiss on the cheek. This childhood training had different effects on them due to the different sexuality socialization processes for males and females. Bob was a sexually active adolescent who bragged about having no sexual problems. He engaged in foreplay not for his enjoyment, but to seduce a woman into having intercourse. When he got an erection, he believed he needed to have an ejaculation, otherwise the woman was a tease and he was angry at her for playing games. Judy felt uncomfortable in sexual interactions, although she engaged in premarital intercourse with several partners. She approached sex with a sense of anxiety and a desire to please the male, not for her own sexual pleasure. She enjoyed kissing, hugging, and caressing because it made her feel cared for and loved. In part, she was compensating for the lack of physical contact and affection she had experienced with her family. On occasion, especially early in a relationship, Judy could be aroused and orgasmic, but did not maintain a sense of sexual comfort and enjoyment.

Judy and Bob's sexual relationship was exciting premaritally and early in the marriage, but became less satisfying after the first year of marriage. Bob had a series of brief extramarital affairs to provide variety and sexual excitement. Judy became involved in a romantic, largely platonic, affair that caused her to consider leaving Bob. She was detoured partly because they now had two young children and she genuinely loved Bob. However, she did not feel loved by him nor sexually attracted to him. The threat of divorce and his reaction to her affair led them to seek marital therapy.

In the course of therapy and in reading about sexuality, it became clear to Bob and Judy how their views about male-female differences, affection, and sexuality had hindered their developing satisfying marital sexuality. Believing at first that he had no sexual problems, Bob became aware that he had an "intimacy" problem. He needed to learn to feel comfortable touching, self-disclosing, and being affectionate with Judy. Bob had to learn to view sexuality as part of the relationship, and not as something separate from it. Most important, he had to realize that sex and affection were good in and of themselves, not as ways of demonstrating masculinity, winning a woman over, or because of being "forbidden fruit." Bob learned to self-disclose, to be emotionally vulnerable, and to cherish emotional and sexuality intimacy in his marriage. Judy had to learn that touching, affection, sensuality, sexuality, intercourse, and orgasm were a continuation of the same feelings and process, rather than viewing affection and sex as two altogether different ways of feeling. Most important, she had to accept that sex was for her as well, not only to please Bob. She needed to give herself permission to be a sexual woman. After eight months of therapy, Bob and Judy had developed positive, integrated attitudes about their marriage and sexual expression. Bob was more comfortable being affectionate and sharing intimate feelings, and Judy was more open to initiating sex and using a variety of arousal techniques in their lovemaking. Judy especially enjoyed and was responsive to multiple stimulation during intercourse.

Judy and Bob resolved to provide their children with a positive sex education, better than what they each had received. In this, they were among a large majority of parents. Over 80 percent of couples want to raise their children with different sexual perceptions. Bob and Judy felt comfortable hugging and kissing not only in the bedroom, but also in the kitchen and living room. In public, they held hands and were affectionate. At first the children were surprised and annoyed at their parents' behavior, especially five-year-old Carol, who said it was "silly" and "gross." Yet both children enjoyed receiving kisses and hugs, especially family hugs.

Although squeamish at first, Judy and Bob could accept their children's awareness and questions. When Brent, their six-year-old, was found playing with his penis in front of Carol, they did not raise the roof and fear he was becoming a sexual deviant. They accepted this as normal childhood sex play, talked to the children about the differences between a penis and vagina, and made the point that one was not better than the other. They made it clear that running around nude outside, forcing other children to take off their clothes as a prank, and touching genitals in public places was not appropriate. They made a clear distinction between sexual play/exploration and sexual coercion/humiliation.

Judy and Bob tried to give their children positive messages about bodies and genitals. They wanted the guidelines to be appropriate, not overly permissive. They did *not* engage in sensual or sexual activity in the presence of their children, encourage the children to touch themselves in front of the picture window, or encourage other children to play sex games. These types of parental behaviors are inappropriate because they intrude on the child's privacy and force sexual expression. Inappropriate parental guidelines cause the child to be hurt and ridiculed by adults and other children. Overly permissive and intrusive handling of sex issues by parents can be just as harmful as overly restrictive and punishing parental behavior.

Contrary to popular mythology, there is *not* a sexual latency period. During the period from six to puberty—between eleven and fourteen for girls and between twelve and sixteen for boys—the child is aware of sexuality issues. Children of seven or eight have boyfriends or girlfriends and talk about who they will marry when they grow up. If a friend's parents divorce, it is not unusual for your child to worry and fear you will divorce.

The most common age for sexual abuse of children is between eight and twelve. Parents need to give clear directions to children about their right to say no to an adult touching their breasts, genitals, or buttocks, or the adult asking or coercing the child to touch him. Most cases of sexual abuse occur with not strangers but with people the child knows. These can include neighbors, church personnel, playground aides, teachers, school personnel, and youth group leaders. Sexual abuse occurs with male as well as female children. The child needs to know that if there is an incident or there are any questions, she can come to you and you will believe and help rather than be angry or blaming.

Intrafamily sexual abuse is a very complex and sensitive topic. Uncles, brothers, stepfathers, in-laws, grandfathers, cousins, and stepbrothers are possible perpetrators of intrafamily sexual abuse. Father-daughter incest is most traumatic because it is such a violation of the trust bond and becomes the "shameful family secret." We encourage fathers to be more involved and affectionate with their children. However, there is a clear line between affectionate touching and sexual abuse. Affectionate touching is nongenital, a sign of caring, and shows respect for the child's person and feelings. Sexual abuse involves genital touching, is done to meet the sexual needs of the perpetrator, and is secretive.

One in three female children and one in seven male children is sexually abused. Most sexual abuse is not violent nor does it involve intercourse. Parents need to talk to their prepubescent child about sexual abuse, and make it clear that she can ask questions or reveal an incident, and that you will listen and emotionally support her.

The preadolescent child is becoming increasingly more aware of himself and will want more privacy when bathing and undressing. At the same time, he is becoming more aware of parents' sexual activity. The child is torn between natural curiosity and embarrassment. Giving both parents and children privacy is the preferred way to deal with this. At the same time, you want to be an approachable and affectionate parent. The single most important guideline is to be an "askable parent." It is crucial to be willing to discuss issues and questions on the child's level of comprehension.

Harold and Susan. Harold and Susan's three children were eleven, nine, and six. A house rule was that mom and dad had private time together and that unless there was something urgent, they were not to be disturbed. One component of private time were talks over a cup of coffee at the kitchen table after dinner. While they were talking, the children did homework, practiced their musical instruments, or played. If the phone rang, one of the children answered and took a message.

Another component of private time was Harold and Susan being in the bedroom. When the door was open, the children knew they could come in and usually did. However, when the door was closed, the children went about their business, took phone messages, and did not interrupt. When the kids were younger, Harold and Susan had put a lock on their bedroom door, and they continued to use it (a lock on the parents' bedroom door is highly recommended). At times, they would go to their bedroom to read. Sometimes they would have intercourse, and other times they would relax, talk, give a back rub, or engage in nondemand pleasuring. Although most of their sexual activity occurred when the children were asleep, they particularly enjoyed sexual experiences when they had more time and energy. In response to their children's curiosity, Harold and Susan said, "We need time together. We love you and enjoy being your mother and father. We love each other and enjoy being married. Sometimes when we are in the bedroom we talk, sometimes we share our love, and sometimes we just want time to ourselves."

Harold and Susan were affectionate with each other and the children. There was no sensual or sexual touching or innuendo in front of the children. Harold and Susan felt their eleven-year-old daughter was at an excellent age for sex education. The school sex program was weak. They had read Sol Gordon's book, *Raising a Child Conservatively in a Sexually Permissive World,* and took a precautionary approach to sex education. Once the daughter and parents got over their initial discomfort, discussing sexual issues from menstruation to contraception to personal values proved worthwhile. Harold and Susan felt better able to handle sexuality discussions with the younger children.

FAMILY SEXUALITY EDUCATION

Talks about sex and privacy are one way for parents to give children informal sex education. The child should be encouraged to partake of many different kinds of such experiences, some formal and some informal. The formal content-based sex education programs offered by schools, the value-oriented sex education programs offered by the church or temple, and the informal sex education of talking with peers are all important. Of crucial importance is family sex education.

Sexuality is an important, integral, complex part of a person's life and must be discussed with respect for that complexity. The old method of sex education included one film in sixth grade, a litany of "don'ts" from the church, a lot of joking, bragging, and myths passed on by the peer group, and a single father-son or mother-daughter talk which emphasized not getting "in trouble.'' This in not the kind of sex education we have in mind, although it is typical of that received by the majority. Ideally, schools would integrate sex education into the curriculum throughout elementary and high school. Churches would give equal weight to positive values regarding sexuality and love as well as sanctions for behavior they judge immoral. Peer groups should be honest and straightforward in discussing sexuality, which would include admitting uncertainty and confusion, and sharing information and experiences, rather than bragging and forcing experimentation in order to keep face. We have a long way to go before we reach this level of sex education.

Family sexuality education is not a one-shot lecture. It is a continuing process of sharing information, exploring feelings and perceptions, and discussing value-oriented issues. Instead of father-son or mother-daughter talks, it includes each parent talking to the child as well as family discussions with both male and female children. More than the simple mechanics of sexuality—physiology, disease, and conception—needs to be covered. Discussion must include feelings, values, and attitudes about a range of topics from masturbation to intercourse, from contraception to sexually transmitted diseases.

There is a tendency to emphasize the harmful because this is what parents fear. Sexual abuse, sexually transmitted diseases, AIDS, sexual assault, and unwanted pregnancies are important issues to deal with, but the initial and primary focus should not be on negatives. You don't want your children to be afraid of sex. You want them to be aware, knowledgeable, and comfortable. As in other areas of life, knowledge is power. A knowledgeable child is more likely to be sexually responsible.

Be sure to orient information to the level of the child's interest and understanding. As in other areas such as how to handle money, or how a car works, you deal with increasing levels of complexity as the child develops. When a seven-year-old asks what inflation means, it is confusing and inappropriate to review Keynesian versus laissez-faire economic theories, so you explain it to her as clearly as you can. In the same way, talk to a seven-year-old on his level when he asks why he gets a "boner" (erection)—don't commence describing the relationship between mental images and erections.

Parents sometimes say that they are ready to answer any question, but that the child doesn't ask. It is your responsibility to establish yourself as an "askable parent." Raise issues and discuss the child's sexual and relationship concerns. You can convey information and perceptions without being intrusive or forcing the child to reveal private matters. Your child needs to feel that she can share information, or ask questions, and that you will listen and respond. Sometimes children will want to have an involved, serious conversation; other times they'll share a joke or observation. Listen to their needs.

The parental message to children should be that sexuality is a positive part of life, that sexual experiences can serve to enhance their lives. Discuss what might hurt them, such as an unwanted pregnancy, being sexually victimized or harassed, rejected in a relationship, feeling inadequate, guilt over masturbation or fantasies, not being comfortable as a male or female. Parents should state as clearly as possible their views regarding masturbation, sex and relationships, and premarital intercourse. The adolescent does not have to—and well may not—share his parents' values, but at least he is aware of them. Discuss your values regarding marriage, family planning, and—if you feel comfortable—marriage and sexuality.

The empirical evidence indicates that the years thirteen to sixteen are the most unhappy time in a person's life. The second most unhappy time is between nineteen and twenty-two. A good portion of the conflict revolves around sexuality. These are periods of experimentation and increased independence. Adolescents and young adults are attempting to develop identities and lives of their own. Not surprisingly, one of the most stressful periods for a couple is when their children are adolescents. Transition periods are difficult for all concerned. You can best handle these by communicating, stating your feelings and limits, and maintaining your role as an approachable parent—someone to turn to if there's trouble, with a question, or to share perceptions and feelings.

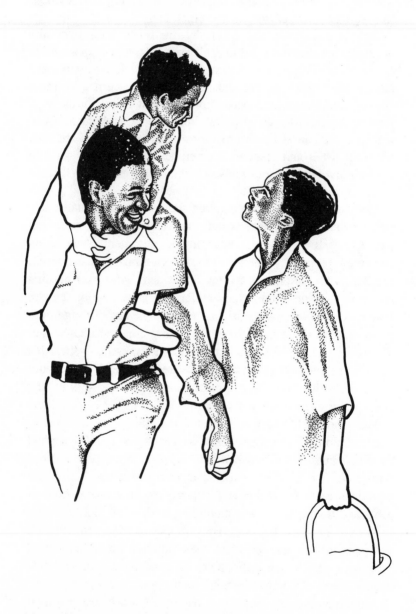

Being affectionate in front of your children and with your children is an important sex education message.

Julia and Mike. Julia and Mike had two children, sixteen-year-old Karen and fourteen-year-old Rob. When the children were younger, nudity was accepted in the home. Julia and Mike were affectionate with each other and the kids. Books about where babies came from, the development of the human body, sexual abuse prevention, and differences between males and females were readily available.

Karen began dating, and there were discussions about how late she would stay out, where she could go, and who she dated. Julia and Mike wanted to do more than set rules. Julia told Karen that she could and should enjoy boys, kissing, and touching. Julia shared her strong feelings that going steady or becoming involved in petting to orgasm was not appropriate at this age. She told Karen that virginity was not the most important thing in the world, but that being good to herself, not getting hurt in a relationship, safeguarding her sexual health, and avoiding pregnancy were important. Mike told Karen he was proud that she was becoming a young woman and that he very much loved her as his daughter. He tried to give her positive messages about males, for, after all, he was once a young man and her younger brother was someone she cared for. He was frank in saying that many boys tried to use girls to "score" and would brag of sexual conquests as a way of proving masculinity. Mike told her that no matter what, her parents loved her and that she could feel free to come to either one with problems or questions.

In addition to individual talks with Karen, Mike and Julia had family discussions that involved Rob. Sexual values, relationships, AIDS, planning children, and marriage were topics. Julia and Mike strongly believed that it was best for their children to delay marriage until young adulthood—twenty-three at the earliest. They wanted the children to have respect for themselves and not to hurt or manipulate others for sexual gain. They tried to give Karen and Rob the same guidelines because they believed in a single standard, not the traditional double standard, for sexuality and relationships. They were honest and practical in making the children aware of the "sex lines and dating games" they would encounter. The children were able to discuss with each other (siblings are important sex educators in the family) their feelings about the double standard and its effects.

To supplement informal discussions, sexuality books were available at the house, and these were read and discussed by both children and adults. For example, a book or pamphlet could serve as the basis for a discussion about various forms of contraception. Mike and Julia mentioned those they had used during marriage, discussing their experiences and weighing positive and negative aspects of each. They encouraged the children to read the chapter on choosing a mate and when to marry. They shared with Karen and Rob their feelings about courtship and marriage. Mike talked about his first marriage. He had married at nineteen, had one child, and was divorced by twenty-two. The children were very interested in this, and Mike discussed what he felt comfortable sharing and chose not to share other things—specifically, that his first wife was six months pregnant when they married.

This points up one of the most difficult dilemmas of the family sexuality approach. The model works best when parents have a good marital and sexual relationship, do not feel guilty about past sexual incidents, and are comfortable sharing personal experiences. Parents can be disappointed or frustrated with the state of their marriage, have had or are having difficult times in their sexual life, may be plagued by feelings of guilt or embarrassment about past behavior, or choose to carefully guard "family secrets."

In deciding what you want to share, recognize and accept your individuality. There is no one right way to educate children sexually. Consider the information and views presented as guidelines, and develop a sex education approach based on your history, relationship, comfort, and values. Be aware that 95 percent of people have had at least one sexual experience that was confusing, guild-inducing, or traumatic, and the majority have had several. Feeling embarrassed or guilty about the past is inappropriate and self-defeating. Guilt serves to lower your self-esteem and make it more difficult to deal with the sex education of your children and present sexual concerns. Each couple needs to decide what of their past behavior, feelings, and attitudes to reveal. Parents should *not* "dump secrets" on children, tell about past sexual escapades, disclose sexual problems, or comment on what arouses them.

It is beneficial for children to realize that parents are individual people. This is especially true of divorced, remarried, or single parents. It is healthy for the child to realize that the adult world has its changes, stresses, and transitions. Growing up with the myth that, once you are married, life remains static and "happy ever after" is not in the child's best interest.

ONGOING SEX EDUCATION

Family sex education is an ongoing process that does not end when children reach eighteen. Both you and they continue to develop and change throughout life. Parents need to realize that children become independent adults who have lives of their own and are responsible for their decisions. Parents feel overly responsible for adult children's marital and sexual adjustment. A parent has a responsibility to give care and attention to the child, but after age eighteen the person is responsible for his behavior. The parent can provide guidance and serve as a resource but may *not* assume responsibility. The best stance is that of a consultant. Parents should not judge the success of their lives by the accomplishments or problems of their children, whether in sexual, vocational, or marital areas.

The aging parent can serve as a model to the adult child that life does not end at sixty. Affection and sexuality can be enjoyed in the sixties, seventies, eighties, and longer. This is one of the best sex education messages you can give.

10
BEING A COUPLE AGAIN

Children are a major life commitment. You are responsible for them for the first eighteen years of their lives. Even after they leave home, parents remain vitally interested in and concerned about their adult children. Raising a child can be one of the most rewarding experiences in a person's life as well as one of the most stressful. Parenting requires immense amounts of time, psychological and physical energy, and commitment. Children need consistent, involved, concerned parents. A common couple trap is to be so involved in the parenting role that you think of yourselves primarily as parents and not as individuals or as a married couple. In an extreme manifestation of this, parents call each other "Mom" and "Dad" and think of themselves in that manner rather than as individual people and spouses.

Throughout the parenting period it is important to remember that you are a person in your own right as well as one-half of a married couple. This attitude, if adopted early in your marriage, sets the stage for a positive transition to being a couple again after the children leave home. We wrote this book when two of our children were young adults and our third child was preparing to leave for college. Especially when the children were younger, we found parenting, to be very satisfying. We especially enjoyed family outings and vacations. We set a priority on taking two weekends a year to go away as a couple without children. This was important when our children were young, but even more so when they were adolescents. We especially remember a week's vacation without the children (they stayed with another family who had children of similar ages and we reciprocated a month later). During that week we had time to swim, sightsee, make love, sit on the beach, and watch sunsets, as well as plan to write our first book together. These experiences helped to keep our marriage vital as well as prepare us for the transition to being a couple again.

When children become young adults and leave home, whether for college, jobs, the service, or training programs, parents experience the "empty nest" syndrome, at one time believed to be a traumatic or at least difficult period of adjustment, especially for women. Recent research and newer conceptualizations challenge this idea. More often, the time is one of individual growth and increased couple intimacy. Couples report heightened marital satisfaction and renewed sexual interest. The empty nest period is certainly a time of transition, but it also can be enhancing, not something to dread.

The norm in our culture is to marry in the mid-twenties and have children soon after. Young adult children usually leave home between the ages of eighteen and twenty-three. Most people become a couple again in their late forties or mid-fifties. Of course, there are wide differences: people may enter this life stage in their late thirties and others not until their sixties. Adult children may return home, sometimes with a grandchild, so that the nest becomes cluttered rather than empty.

Most couples will have as much, or more, time together as they spent parenting. A major guideline is to be aware, while you are still actively functioning in the parental role, of the prime importance of the marital bond. People who realize that first they are individuals, then a married couple, and then parents, do best at those roles. Those who value their individuality and couple bond are more satisfied with their lives and, in the long run, are better parents. Do not make being a couple subservient to being a parent, even when children are young.

The most important relationship in a family is the husband-wife bond. If that bond is vital, it makes parenting easier and is in the best interest of the children.

Being a couple again is an important transition for your marital and sexual relationship. Like other transitions, it can be a time of increased growth and satisfaction, yet it involves potential traps and risks. The more aware you are of these opportunities and problems, the better your decision-making and ability to adopt positive coping strategies. This is a time to revitalize the marital and sexual bond.

Alice and Tom. Alice and Tom, a couple in their late forties, very much enjoyed raising their three children. Ralph was twenty-six, married, and started on his career. Andi was a senior in college and Jim had just moved out of the house and begun a training program in forestry management. For the first time in twenty-six years there were no children living at home, although they would visit on weekends and during vacations. The adjustment was somewhat more difficult for Alice than Tom, since she had been more involved on a day-to-day basis. Eight years before, she had begun preparing herself for this transition by returning to school and completing her degree in computer programming. She had recently received a major job promotion to systems analyst.

Tom and Alice welcomed the increasing independence and maturity of their children. It allowed them time and freedom to pursue their interests. Alice became more heavily invested in her job and was elected an officer in her professional organization. Tom had greater opportunity to pursue his hobbies. With the financial burden lifted, and two substantial incomes, they were able to indulge themselves. One of their first purchases was camping equipment oriented for two people instead of a family. They found it freeing to no longer have to schedule weekend trips and vacations around children's school and extra-curricular activities. Although Tom and Alice were not particularly verbal or feeling-oriented in their couple communication style, they very much enjoyed doing things together and sharing

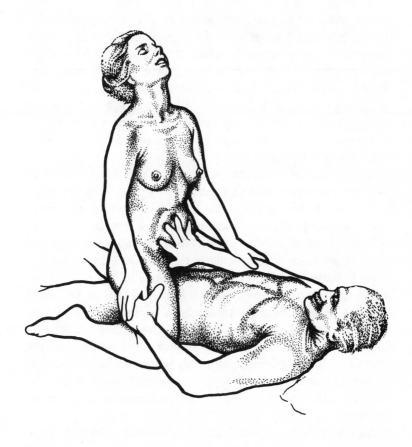

Take advantage of the time and privacy to experiment with prolonged intercourse and multiple stimulation.

outdoor experiences. Tom bought some long desired photography equipment. Alice was not expert in photography, but did enjoy accompanying him on picture-taking trips. She herself was freer to travel to seminars on computer management, and had a sense of increased professional competence.

No longer concerned about interruptions from children, their sexual relationship was more adventuresome and spontaneous. They discovered "nooners" were a particularly exciting sexual experience, especially after years of relegating sex to a late night activity. Their lovemaking became more creative and flexible. Alice could walk around the house in a bra and panties—or nude, if she desired. Tom experienced a renewed sense of sexual desire as they had sex in the den, necked on the living room couch, made love in the guest bedroom, and slept there through the night.

Alice especially enjoyed prolonged sexual pleasuring. Not having to worry about being interrupted by phone calls, children making noise, or knocks on the door ignited her sexual desire. Alice would suggest taking a ten-minute break from the pleasuring to have a glass of wine and talk. When they returned to genital stimulation, Alice was particularly receptive and responsive.

Tom enjoyed the opportunity to be sexual in different places, including taking advantage of camping weekends to be sexual outdoors. They would go wilderness camping and make love under the stars. Tom also relished creative sexual scenarios at home. He enjoyed doing sexual play in one room and having intercourse in a different room. Tom accompanied Alice to her conventions and used these opportunities to compare Hilton and Marriott hotel rooms to see which promoted a more sexual environment.

Alice and Tom continued active interest in parenting. They enjoyed their adult children coming home for Thanksgiving and other occasions. Tom and Alice also visited them on their "turf," an implicit acknowledgement that the children were independent adults with lives of their own. Alice and Tom talked with their children about a variety of matters, including sexual issues. Tom was particularly pleased that Andi and Jim sought his advice about housing and financial decisions. Tom and Alice gave guidance when it was requested, without forcing their views. They recognized that Ralph, Andi, and Jim were adults responsible for their own lives. They loved and were concerned about their children, but did not assume the burden of responsibility for their successes and problems. They adopted the role of consultant to their adult children, and did not offer advice unless it was requested.

DIFFICULT TRANSITIONS

Not everyone will make such a positive adjustment to being a couple again. Problems occur when couple interaction has centered chiefly around children. With this topic of conversation gone, the couple finds they have little to talk about. An extreme example is parents who put pressure on adult children to have a baby so that they can have a grandchild to focus on. They need a child-oriented role as grandparents because they refuse to interact as a couple.

Not having anything to communicate and finding that there are few shared interests can be a rude awakening. The couple is afraid to admit that this is the state of their marital relationship, because to do so could entail a move toward divorce with a loss of the security of more than twenty years of married life. The couple who deny that there is a problem will not put energy into rebuilding the relationship, so it will continue to stagnate. Such empty nest marriages are mediocre at best and can disintegrate into lonely, bitter relationships. A sexual dysfunction such as an erection problem, inability to reach orgasm, and/or inhibited sexual desire for one or both partners, is likely to develop. Lack of sexual desire generalizes to avoidance of any affectionate interchange which accelerates the process of resentment and alienation.

Couples who admit they have grown apart and are facing serious problems can mobilize their resources and energy toward rebuilding a sharing, communicative, and sexual marriage. The vitality of a marital bond can and often does dissipate under the stresses and strains of raising teenagers. Facing this reality allows the couple to focus on rebuilding their marital bond.

With children gone, there is an excellent opportunity to deal with each other and set the stage for a satisfying marital and sexual relationship into the sixties and beyond.

Donna and Jeff. Donna and Jeff were a struggling couple who had become so used to practical problems and adolescent hassles that they did not know what to do when they were a couple again. Donna had three children from her first marriage, which ended when her husband died in a car accident. Four years later she married Jeff, who had two children from a first marriage and one from a second. Jeff's children stayed with them on an intermittent basis. Stepfamilies are not, and should not try to be, a replica of the traditional nuclear family. Blended families have their unique stresses as well as their unique strengths and learning opportunities.

Donna and Jeff found adolescent crises draining. They would fight about child management problems, finances, practical matters like who was going to clean up after the dog, or their unhappiness with each other. Donna would feel herself becoming depressed, which coincided with Jeff's drinking too much. It seemed anticlimactic for the children to be gone and to have a relatively stress-free home life. For a time they considered becoming more involved in their adult children's marriages and in taking care of grandchildren, but wisely decided not to. Although they were willing to help on a temporary basis and in a crisis, they realized that too much intervention would interfere with the adult children finding their own solutions.

Jeff and Donna were uneasy being with each other. During the previous ten years they'd engaged in relatively few couple activities. Intercourse had decreased to less than once a month. The first step in revitalizing their couple bond was to accept the reality of the situation. Instead of being frightened and fearful, they resolved to make a good faith effort.

They decided to go on a week's vacation which turned into a second honeymoon. They enjoyed the trip and, more importantly, used the time to share feelings and reestablish their sexual relationship. On the last day of vacation, Donna sat the two of them down. She wanted a commitment to continue being affectionate and to keep their sexual relationship on track rather than their falling into old habits and ignoring each other except when there was a conflict.

They settled into the routine of jobs, housework, social activities, contact with children and grandchildren, and neighborhood meetings. They did reserve two evenings a week for couple activities. Sometimes they worked together around the house. Other times they went to a movie, had a sexual date, watched TV, went for a walk. Intercourse frequency was one or two times per week. They did not strive for the perfect marriage described in magazine articles. They wanted a marriage that met their needs. Donna and Jeff were individualists who resented the notion that marriage was supposed to be communicative and loving twenty-four hours a day, seven days a week. What was important was knowing that they could depend on each other, enjoy the other's company, cuddle on the couch, and make love.

Are there marriages based on children or security in which it is not possible to resurrect intimate feelings? We've seen a good many couples who have lost touch with one another, or perhaps never had an intimate relationship, for whom sex was infrequent or nonexistent. The marriage was functional in meeting companionate, financial, and/or practical needs. Although needs for emotional intimacy and sexual fulfillment were not met, these needs were not high priority for them. There were couples who stayed married and enjoyed the marriage even though there was little or no sexual satisfaction. These couples chose to focus on other aspects of their lives which were fulfilling.

GUIDELINES FOR BEING A COUPLE AGAIN

Couples who value intimate, sexual expression can implement the following guidelines.

1. Acknowledge that you are going through a major transition.
2. Be aware that you have different interests and needs than when you first married.

3. Accept that your relationship and sexual interests/needs have changed during these years. Sexuality needs to be more cooperative and interactive, and involve more than intercourse.

4. Commit to put time and psychological energy into your marriage.

5. Be open and direct during sexual play. Sensuality, mutual genital stimulation, and multiple stimulation will increase sexual satisfaction.

6. Be aware of yourselves as sexual people and as a sexual couple, separate from your parental role.

Working on your relationship requires a genuine commitment to communicate feelings, make clear and direct requests, be open to your spouse's needs and desires, and, most important, to live in the present rather than to be shackled with disappointments, resentments, and regrets over missed opportunities of the past. One of the worst traps to fall into is the "if only" type of thinking. Focus your psychological and sexual energy on the present and future.

For many couples, the major roadblock to revitalizing the sexual bond is their history. You cannot be married to someone for more than twenty years and not have memories of hurt, anger, disappointment, and resentment. The question is whether you are going to allow those to control your life and marriage. In his clinical work, Barry asks each spouse to make a list of incidents that still grate on them. Then he asks each to state what might be done in the present to alleviate past feelings or to change the present situation. The most common request is for the spouse to acknowledge the feelings and offer a genuine apology.

ALTERNATIVES TO A REVITALIZED MARITAL BOND

If a couple finds that this approach to revitalizing the marital bond is not acceptable or productive, they have several alternatives. One is to realize that their marriage does not and will not meet their needs, and separate or divorce. A second is to keep the security of the marriage, but to develop a more independent and autonomous life in which some needs—perhaps including sexual needs—are met outside the marriage. A third alternative is to become involved in the grandparent role and relate to each other as grandparents. The latter role is satisfactory to many couples, although we strongly caution not to put pressure on adult children to produce grandchildren to fulfill your needs. Another alternative is to continue as you have been. There is more to life than emotional intimacy and sexual satisfaction. Friendships, job satisfaction, hobbies, extended family contact, and social, religious, and community activities provide major satisfactions. Your marriage can continue to meet companionship and security needs.

There is no such thing as a perfect marriage. Each individual and couple has their own needs and values. You are the only one who can determine what is in your best interest. Your decisions and adjustments will probably be somewhat different, or in some cases, such as those that follow, entirely different from our guidelines.

Rose and Bill. Rose and Bill have been married thirty-three years. Their youngest child left home to be married at twenty-one. Their three children live in the same neighborhood and they have two grandchildren. Bill and Rose had an inactive sex life for much of their marriage and have not engaged in intercourse for the past ten years. They are involved in their jobs and church activities. The entire family gathers for Sunday dinner, and this family ritual is highly valued by Rose and Bill. They regularly babysit for their grandchildren and take the grandchildren with them on summer vacation. For Bill and Rose, this is a satisfying marriage and life.

Although they chose a marital style that is contrary to most of the guidelines of this book, it is one that satisfies their needs and is an excellent choice for them. Every couple is unique; there is no one "right" way to attain psychological well-being or marital satisfaction.

Let us consider a couple who attempted to follow our guidelines and found they did not meet their needs.

Nick and Jean. Nick and Jean had two children. When at nineteen their younger daughter went to work in another town, they found themselves, in their late forties and having been married twenty-three years, feeling awkward about being a couple again. They believed the missing element was communication, and attended a marriage enrichment weekend and read books on couple communication. They purchased one of the zanier sex manuals and tried some of the more esoteric techniques and positions. Children and friends supported these efforts to revitalize the marital relationship. Nick and Jean were perceived by friends as a model of a successful "couple again."

After eighteen months, they continued to be dissatisfied with their marital and sexual relationship. After the initial thrill of trying a new sexual technique, they found little pleasure in their sex. They were baffled and decided to seek professional marriage therapy. The clinician tried to help them gain a deeper understanding of themselves and their relationship.

After three months of therapy, the clinician asked them to focus on an issue they had been avoiding for two years—the possibility that they had grown so far apart that it really was not possible to revitalize their marriage. Couples sometimes badly stretch their marital bond, but it remains intact. Once a marital bond is broken, i.e., the respect, trust, and intimacy is destroyed and they no longer think of themselves as a couple, it is very difficult to resurrect. Nick and Jean had to face a hard choice between holding onto a marriage that would never be more than mediocre or taking a major risk and going their separate ways. It was Jean who decided she wanted more out of life than a secure but unfulfilling marriage. She initiated a separation with Nick's reluctant agreement. The therapist continued to see Nick to help him work through his feelings of disappointment and adjusting to being single again. Although the children understood intellectually that their parents would be happier living alone or remarrying, they had great emotional difficulty accepting the decision. That's not unusual; adult children find it difficult to accept parents having lives of their own and undergoing changes, especially changes in their marital relationship.

CLOSING THOUGHTS

The transition to being a couple again can result in revitalization of the marriage and a new sense of freedom and spontaneity in the sexual relationship, or it can cause personal, marital, and sexual dissatisfaction, with major changes in one's life.

Although couples are anxious and unsure about returning to the couple-again stage, it can be a period of growth in intimacy and sexuality. Opportunities for privacy, increased couple time, and the development of new individual and couple interests is exciting. You may have less inhibited, more creative, and intimate sex. Having adolescent or young adult children in the home is confining and inhibits sensual and sexual expression. It feels delicious, if not illicit, to prance around your home with seductive clothing on—or off—and make love in the den, living room, or even kitchen without fear of children coming home unexpectedly. The couple who learn and grow through this transition have a solid foundation for their aging years. Being a couple again can be satisfying personally, maritally, and sexually. As we write this book, we look forward to this stage in our marriage.

11
SEX AFTER SIXTY

You are a sexual person from the day you're born until the day you die. A couple in good physical health can function sexually into their sixties, seventies, eighties, and longer. We will explore how the couple can develop an understanding of, and positive attitudes toward, the physiological, psychological, marital, and sexual transitions that occur after sixty.

Until recently, the older person consulting a physician or marriage therapist for advice about his sexual functioning would be faced with an embarrassed laugh and told either to leave sex to younger people or not to worry since, when sexual functioning wanes, there is nothing you can do. Now, if you consult a well-trained professional, you'll find a wealth of information and specific suggestions on making sexuality a positive, integral part of the aging process. Recent research has found that if couples (1) understand and accept changes in sexual functioning that occur with aging, (2) maintain good health and are aware of possible sexual side effects of medication, and (3) have positive attitudes and are open to a broad-based approach to sexual expression, their sexual relationships can and will be satisfying.

ATTITUDES TOWARD SEX AND AGING

As with other aspects of human sexuality, the process involves awareness, acceptance, and communication. The more this occurs through the middle years, the easier it will be to transfer positive attitudes, feelings, and behavior to your later years. Key elements in couple sexual functioning are acceptance of your body image as an aging person and having an interested and responsive partner. A couple with a history of regular and satisfying sexual relations has a solid basis for continuing pleasurable sexual expression into their older years.

One of the most harmful myths is that males should save their ejaculations because they only have so much semen, and if they overuse it when younger there will be none left. The facts are just the opposite. Men do not run out of ejaculations, nor do women run out of orgasms. The more regular the sexual expression, the easier and more comfortable is continuing it. Sex is a natural physiological function and, as with walking, dancing, or playing tennis, the old adage is true: "Use it or lose it."

Our culture idolizes youth and beauty. One of the worst assumptions is that sexual attractiveness depends on a woman having firm thighs and breasts or a man being slim and muscular. If your image of sexuality is based on youthful physical characteristics, you are setting yourself up to feel rejected and sexually unattractive as you age. Your sense of sexual attractiveness is better based on enjoying sensations of touch, being comfortable with your body, enjoying your partner and her sensitivities, giving and receiving pleasure, and integrating sexuality into your self-image. Sex is not just intercourse and orgasm, nor does sexuality reside primarily in your genitals. Sexuality is an expression of feelings, body image, self-concept, intimate sharing, and a sense of pleasure—it is integral to who you are. This concept of sexuality is as applicable to the forty- or seventy-year-old as to the twenty-year-old. It forms a healthy basis for lifelong sexuality and facilitates acceptance of a positive body image as you age. Sexuality is not facilitated by striving to regain youth and beauty, but belongs to you as a person and is an integral part of your couple bond.

In Barry's college course Human Sexual Behavior, there is a lecture on sex and aging with a film showing a couple in their sixties engaging in a series of pleasurable sexual interactions. After initial anxiety and discomfort, students find this class session a highlight of the course. Realizing that an aging couple can enjoy sexual expression, continuing to learn and share, is a comforting concept. It removes the pressure to know and experience everything by the time the student reaches twenty-one. The idea that college students have fifty years of sexual functioning and experiences to look forward to is liberating. There is sex after college! The view of sexuality as a lifelong process of giving and receiving pleasure facilitates acceptance of sexuality and the aging process.

This is certainly a different view of sex and aging than the stereotypic presentation of the dirty old man and the dried up, asexual woman. Sex among older people is standard fare for the comedian's repertoire. This perception comes from younger people's anxiety about, and inability to view, older adult figures as sexual people. In an informal survey taken in the Human Sexual Behavior class, only one in four students could imagine their parents having sexual intercourse and only one in twelve could imagine their grandparents being sexually active. Young adults are so used to parents and grandparents telling them not to have sex that it is hard for them to imagine parents and grandparents engaging in sex, much less deriving pleasure from it. Older adults, whether in the middle years or senior citizens, can improve the image of sex and aging by acknowledging that they are, and enjoy being, sexual.

An extreme example of the denial of sexuality may occur when a parent enters a nursing home. Their adult children might insist that there be no affectionate touching or sexual contact with other residents. The major reason for this irrational position is that adult children cannot accept, since they have always denied, their parents affectional and sexual needs. This is detrimental to those who reside in nursing homes; it denies their right to privacy and the comfort of human contact. The need for human contact is vital from the time you're a baby through the middle years and into your sunset years.

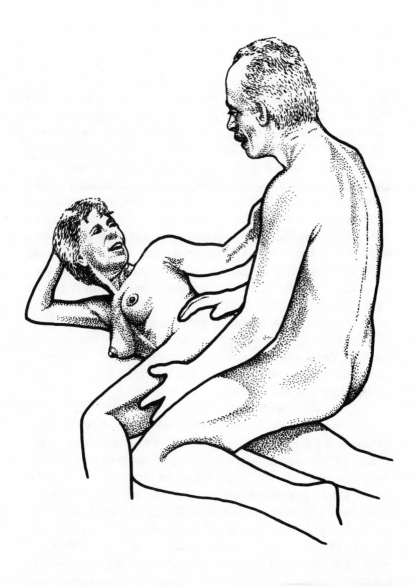

Appreciate a relaxed non-demand approach to touching, sensuality and sexuality. You can be sexual into your sixties, seventies, eighties and beyond.

Let us consider a couple who enjoyed their marital and sexual life throughout the middle years and made an easy transition to sexuality and aging.

Pat and Daryl. Pat and Daryl were married when he was twenty-three and she twenty-one. They had three children, the last born when he was twenty-nine and she twenty-seven. Pat and Daryl valued their couple bond and throughout the marriage put energy into communicating, experimenting, and building feelings of caring and intimacy. At fifty, with their adult children living away from home, the transition to being a couple again was smooth. They enjoyed having more time for themselves and each other. They valued the other's sexual interests and needs. More than half their pleasure came from the spouse's feelings and responses. The "give to get" pleasure principle worked well in their marriage. In sexual interactions that were mediocre or not successful—about one in ten, which is normal for a sexually functional couple—they accepted this and laughed about it rather than blaming, being angry, or feeling guilty about not satisfying the spouse. They sometimes had sex two times in three days or went for a week without intercourse. They accepted this variability without worrying about their normality or performance.

As Daryl approached sixty, he found he needed Pat's direct penile stimulation in order to obtain an erection. She felt comfortable using a variety of techniques to arouse him, from gently massaging the shaft to putting his penis in her mouth to stroking the glans with one hand and massaging his testicles with the other. They were adept and comfortable with a side-by-side (scissors) intercourse position as well as the position where the woman's leg is over the man's and he enters from the side. In these two positions, Pat found it easier to insert his penis when he was not fully erect. As intercourse progressed arousal built as did the erection.

They kept a bottle of Aloe Vera handy to use for additional vaginal lubrication if needed. Daryl became comfortable using spittle as a lubricant. They had learned in their thirties that nondemand pleasuring and multiple stimulation were the keys to sexual arousal, knowledge that held them in good stead for the aging years. Daryl and Pat felt at ease occasionally taking a break to sip a glass of wine, talk about feelings, or share sexual fantasies. This pleasurable, nondemand interaction provided a fresh and varied dimension to their love play and allowed sexual arousal to gradually build.

Throughout the marriage, Pat had been multiorgasmic in many of their sexual encounters. As she aged, her muiltiorgasmic response pattern began to change. She had typically been orgasmic five to seven times, and now she experienced one, two, or three orgasms. At times, she would not be orgasmic. She did not want to force herself or have Daryl push her to have an orgasm. She respected the rhythm of her sexual needs instead of demanding that her body respond as it had when she was forty-five.

Daryl found he desired to ejaculate two of the three times they had intercourse. Once or twice he pushed himself to ejaculate even when he did not have a need, and though he was able to, it was not pleasurable and a week passed before he desired to have intercourse again. Daryl decided he would ejaculate only when he felt the sexual need instead of forcing himself to reach orgasm each time. He explained to Pat that sex was good for him even when he did not ejaculate. Some men feel they achieve a sexual sensation similar to orgasm even though they don't ejaculate. Daryl's experience was that sex was pleasurable, but that he was not orgasmic.

Daryl and Pat learned to accept and enjoy intercourse even though one or both were not orgasmic. Pleasure and intimacy are the prime motives for sex, not orgasm. Orgasm is not always necessary, nor is it the criterion to measure whether a sexual experience was satisfying.

At times, Pat and Daryl engaged in affectionate touching and sensual pleasuring that were pleasant but not highly arousing. This pattern developed early in the marriage when every two months they would set aside an evening that was devoted to pleasuring and nondemand experiences which would not end in intercourse and orgasm. This formed the basis for functional and pleasurable sexuality in their sixties. The strategies and techniques used by Pat and Daryl are well worth considering in your marriage, whether you are in your thirties, fifties, or seventies. The nondemand concepts advocated throughout this book reach their fruition in sexual expression after sixty.

ISSUES IN SEX AND AGING

One of the most harmful myths is the belief that if a couple has had sexual problems in the middle years, their sex life will necessarily deteriorate as they age. For the aware and motivated couple, the opposite can occur. A man who has consistently been an early ejaculator can achieve ejaculatory control as part of the aging process. In the older male, ejaculation becomes a single-phase response which facilitates development of ejaculatory control.

With a lessened pressure for rapid sexual performance, both men and women can gain greater enjoyment with prolonged sensual and sexual stimulation. The key elements for effective sexual functioning are nondemand pleasuring, an intimate relationship, the enjoyment of a broad range of sensual and sexual stimulation techniques, understanding and accepting physiological changes, accepting your body image, awareness of altered patterns of sexual response, communicating these to your spouse, engaging in multiple stimulation, and working together to integrate changes into your couple sexual style. This can be adopted by an older couple even if the sexual experiences of their younger and middle years were not satisfying.

The most enjoyable clinical case Barry ever had involved a couple in their sixties who had been married thirty-seven years. Their marriage had been good in spite of a terribly dysfunctional sexual relationship. They'd read about sex therapy and self-referred themselves to see if anything had changed since their abortive attempt at sex counseling with a physician twenty years before. This couple proceeded through sex therapy just like "in the book." The nongenital and genital pleasuring exercises caused an awakening in their bodies; with two months of therapy, she was orgasmic for the first time in her life. Even more than orgasmic response was the pleasure experienced in sharing a passion felt for years but just now expressed.

ILLNESS AND DEATH OF A SPOUSE

An extremely sensitive issue arises when one spouse becomes ill and/or is dying. Death is even more of a taboo subject in our society than is sexuality. When you combine the subjects of aging, sex, and death, you have an enormous amount of myth, anxiety, confusion, and misunderstanding. The more aware and knowledgeable a couple is, the easier it will be to deal with this most difficult and complex area. The appropriate time to think about and discuss these issues is when both people are healthy, not in the middle of a crisis.

What happens when one spouse becomes extremely, and perhaps terminally ill? The seriously ill person continues to have needs for affection and touching. To withdraw this contact is to further depress and, in a manner, to abandon the spouse. Contrary to popular myth, affectionate and sensual contact is both possible, enjoyable, and psychologically healthy for the ailing person. Even if sexual intercourse is not desired, most ill people, and especially terminally ill people, desire the caring that is demonstrated by touch.

One factor in sexual adjustment to the spouse's illness involves feelings and attitudes toward masturbation. The majority of married men and women occasionally masturbate. Masturbation is a normal and healthy sexual behavior at any time in a person's life, but especially during a spouse's illness. A harmful myth is that an adult masturbating is regressive behavior and a sign of senility. Masturbation for a widow or widower is an affirmation of sexuality and is a perfectly normal and appropriate means of sexual expression.

Couples are well advised to discuss, while they are still healthy, their feelings about dating or remarriage when a spouse dies. This is a value-oriented question each individual must decide for herself. The spouse does not have to be in interminable mourning and deny her needs for companionship, affection, and sex. It has been said that women mourn and men replace after a spouse dies. We believe that both men and women need to mourn, and that afterward both need to consider how to organize their lives. Deciding to be asexual is one alternative open to the survivor. Remarrying, having sex with other partners, masturbating, and being emotionally involved but not sexually active with other people are alternatives to consider.

Rita and John. Rita and John were in their late sixties and had been married forty-three years when Rita contracted cancer. She undertook surgery but unfortunately it was too late, the cancer had spread through the lymph glands. During her last year of life, Rita and John engaged in sexual intercourse, usually at her initiation, about once a month. There were many experiences involving back rubs and lying together and holding. John used masturbation as a sexual outlet, and although not explicitly discussed, this was understood and accepted by both.

Physical closeness was important as they prepared for her impending death. Two months before she died, sexual intercourse became unpleasant for Rita, but affection and emotional intimacy were desired and continued. Physical closeness facilitated greater sharing of feelings, which included sadness, love, grief, anger, and resignation. This helped Rita better prepare for and accept her death. John was able to express his feelings as well as do the essential cooking and cleaning to keep the house functional. Holding and talking helped him deal with the grieving process people experience when a spouse dies. Engaging in anticipatory grieving while the spouse is alive is emotionally painful, yet psychologically worthwhile, for both people.

When John began a relationship with another woman fourteen months after Rita's death, he had difficulty keeping an erection and having intercourse. This is to be expected since even though he regularly masturbated he had not attempted intercourse for almost a year and a half. As with any other physical activity— swimming for example—there is a need to get back in practice.

This common phenomenon has been labeled the "widower's syndrome." John did not overreact to his temporary erectile disorder. He continued to engage in sexual activity that emphasized nondemand pleasuring and manual and oral stimulation. Instead of avoiding sexual contact, which would have led to performance anxiety and eroded his sexual confidence, he continued to engage in pleasure-oriented sexual expression. As his sexual comfort and involvement increased, so did his erectile functioning. Eventually, he developed a satisfying sexual relationship, including intercourse, with the new partner. John did not make comparisons between his marriage and this relationship. The best way to approach sexuality and aging, especially in a new relationship, is a positive one. Focus on the new relationship, don't make comparisons with the past.

Juanita and Roy. Juanita and Roy, a couple in their middle forties, had two teenage children. Juanita's parents were alive and married, Roy's mother, a widow, shared her house with a woman friend. Roy and Juanita were committed to keeping their marriage sexually satisfying and to raising their children in a sexually healthy environment. They looked forward to continuing sexual expression into their sixties and beyond.

Juanita's parents were from the old school of thought which held that sex, politics, and religion were three topics never discussed. They were not affectionate and had moved to separate bedrooms twenty years before. Not only were they not a good model of an over-sixty couple, but Juanita doubted that sex had ever been satisfying for her mother. When her father made a comment that Juanita and Roy would eventually lose their affectionate manner, they were not argumentative but simply said that they looked forward to being affectionate their entire married lives, including when they were grandparents. Their teenage children heard that conversation and understood their parents' message.

Roy's mother had been a widow for over ten years. Roy made it a point to tell her that he would accept her dating or remarrying and that he would not consider this disloyal to the memory of his father. Roy encouraged his mother to be social and to do what would make her happy. She did not remarry, although she was active in social groups and had male friends. She also confided to Juanita that she felt sexual urges and masturbated to reduce tension, but asked Juanita not to tell Roy. She did ask whether Juanita felt that an old lady masturbating was perverse. Juanita assured her mother-in-law that this was normal and healthy, and shared that she occasionally masturbated— not because she did not love Roy or was not sexually satisfied with him but to enjoy self-pleasuring as an additional sexual experience. Juanita realized that widows have fewer choices of available men, and urged her mother-in-law to avoid entering into a caretaking relationship.

Roy and Juanita had positive attitudes toward middle-years sexuality and were establishing a base for sexual functioning in their later years. They accepted their aging and the aging of others and were aware that needs for touching, affection, sensuality, and sexuality would extend throughout their lifetime.

IMAGES OF SEX AND AGING

The negative image of sex and aging is based on the myth that sexual expression is an animalistic, uncontrollable need associated with behaviors such as seeking out younger women or sexually molesting children. These images are exclusively associated with males, as if aging females were sexual neuters. This conceptualization of sex and aging is grossly inaccurate. Sexual abuse incidents involve less than 2 percent of males and are associated primarily with adolescent and young adult men. More to the point, the need for sexual contact is neither animalistic nor inappropriate, but the result of a natural physiological function and a psychological need for touch and caring.

Sexual feelings and expression are normal throughout the life span for both women and men. Touching, affection, sensuality, and sexuality are important in the sixties, seventies, eighties, and beyond. Other sources of pleasure and satisfaction are less available in later years. A person may not be as robust physically or no longer has job satisfaction or monetary rewards. Couples have the opportunity to lead a less hectic, less performance-oriented life. They can appreciate a relaxed, nondemand approach to living, including touching, sensuality, and sexuality. Our society needs to accept that touching/affection and sexual arousal/orgasm are normal and appropriate for aging women and men.

The more a couple understands physiological changes in their bodies, the better prepared they'll be to adapt their sexual functioning. The most important changes affecting the male are that he no longer has the need to ejaculate at each sexual intercourse, that his erection will take longer to develop, he'll need more direct penile stimulation, and his erection will be less firm. After ejaculation, there may be one, two, or more days before he will again respond to sexual stimulation. The female typically experiences lessened vaginal lubrication and takes longer to become aroused and reach orgasm. Changes are gradual rather than dramatic, beginning between forty-five and sixty-five. Contrary to popular myth, changes affect men more than women. There are tremendous individual differences in the rate at which these changes occur. It is crucial to be aware, to accept, and to communicate about changes in physiological function. They do not have to lead to a decrease in sexual feeling or satisfaction.

When couples stop being sexual, over 95 percent of the time it is the male who no longer wants to be sexual. Couples do not discuss this—it is a unilateral decision. He decides, because of erectile dysfunction or inhibited sexual desire, that sex is just too difficult and not worth it. The male's double standard assumptions ultimately sabotage his sexual functioning and the couple's sexual relationship. Men and women who are aware and open to viewing sexuality in a broader-based, more interactive and pleasure-oriented manner can continue to have satisfying sensual and sexual experiences throughout their lives.

CLOSING THOUGHTS

As you age, a variety of physical, psychological, relational, and situational changes occur. These changes have both direct and indirect effects on your sexual functioning. The more you understand the changes, communicate about, and accept them, the easier it will be to maintain a satisfying sexual relationship into your sixties, seventies, eighties, and beyond.

12
ENHANCING SEXUAL DESIRE

At the beginning of a relationship, it is natural to feel taken by and sexually desirous of your new partner. The sense of novelty, illicitness, and romantic ecstasy which fills the first few weeks or months of a relationship is an experience not to be missed. However, sexual desire that comes from romantic ecstasy seldom lasts as long as two years and is likely to disappear after six months. That doesn't mean you've fallen out of love or you no longer find your partner attractive. It does mean that the initial sexual rush from romantic love is over. Seldom does it last until marriage, much less a year into the marriage.

Intimacy is the enduring source of sexual desire in marriage. The immediate stimuli for sexual desire are more specific and erotic. Stimuli for sexual desire can be a sexual dream or fantasy, a sexually-oriented movie or an erotic passage in a novel, an attractive or seductive person on the street, your partner initiating and being aroused, an affectionate or sensual interchange, or anticipation of a special opportunity to be sexual. Contrary to popular thinking, long intervals between sexual opportunities do not build "horniness." It is regularity of sexual expression that builds and reinforces sexual desire. Like other types of physical activity—walking, biking, swimming—the person who has a regular rhythm of activity anticipates, enjoys, and values it. Anticipating, enjoying, and valuing sexuality is the best way to establish and maintain sexual desire.

The approach we advocate is different from the movie and musical images of sexuality. In the movies there is instant chemical attraction, a slow tantalizing buildup, and then an explosion of overwhelming, overpowering sexual ecstasy. After seeing an R-rated movie, Barry's clients ask why their sex life can't be like that. The Hollywood scenario sells movies, but makes for poor real-life sex, especially sexual desire in an ongoing marriage. The kind of sex that sells in movies is destructive to marital sexuality because it creates unrealistic and self-defeating expectations.

What are the sources of sexual desire in an ongoing marriage? The most important are positive feelings about the spouse and past experiences that build anticipation for future sexual scenarios. The components of sexual desire are feeling good about yourself as a sexual person, believing that you deserve sexual pleasure, and anticipating the sexual experience. Other sources of sexual desire include intimate feelings toward your spouse, affectionate and sensual touching both inside and outside the bedroom, success on the job or athletic field, or successful completion of a project. Sex can also be anticipated as a tension reducer after a hard day; movie, fantasy, or the sight of someone attractive may promote desire; sex may be a way to compensate for a defeat in another area of life; and taking a vacation and having the freedom and privacy to act on sexual feelings may stimulate them. Sexual desire can and should come from a number of sources, especially feelings and anticipation.

BLOCKS TO SEXUAL DESIRE

Occasional lack of sexual desire is an almost universal phenomenon for both women and men although it's true men would not admit it. Stresses such as illness, job pressure, depression, lack of sleep, worry about children, grieving, money pressures, and anxiety result in lessened sexual desire. This is temporary—when the stress lifts desire returns. Low sexual desire is a

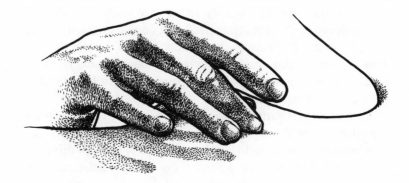

Anticipating, and valuing touching and sexuality is the best way to maintain sexual desire.

problem only when it extends over a long period of time and causes problems in the couple's relationship.

Inhibited sexual desire—the technical, clinical term for this problem—is the most common complaint of couples seeking sexual therapy. Approximately 33 percent of married women and 15 percent of married men complain of inhibited sexual desire. Over time desire problems become more severe and chronic. Couples argue about the lack of sexual frequency, and conflicts over initiation and rejection loom larger. These degenerate into power struggles filled with name-calling and blaming.

Couples plagued with inhibited sexual desire focus on the wrong issue. They emphasize frequency; one partner tries to convince the other to have intercourse. A more productive focus would be on improving quality rather than quantity. Inhibited sexual desire is best conceptualized as a couple problem, which avoids putting the pressure, blame, and stigma on one partner. This is not to shift blame, but to say that if sex is to be functional and pleasurable the two people need to be a team in developing a couple sexual style.

Even when one partner—usually the woman—reports primary inhibited sexual desire (which means she never thought of sex as a positive element in life and always had a low sex drive), it is a couple's task to develop a satisfying sexual relationship. We encourage couples to seek professional therapy for problems of inhibited sexual desire to help them break the pattern of blame and guilt and learn to be an intimate sexual team. More than other sexual problems, inhibited sexual desire brings out the worst reactions in the partner, which further undermines the marriage. The spouse with higher desire sometimes blames himself, but most often blames the partner. He accuses her of being inhibited and tries to convince or coerce her to be sexual. He might threaten to leave or have an affair. When it's the women with higher desire, she sees his lack of interest as a personal rejection or as a sign of her lack of attractiveness. There is suspicion that the spouse is having an affair. The self-blame and frustration is turned against the partner. Especially harmful is an attack on his masculinity, or her femininity. These reactions are self-defeating and serve to exacerbate the problem.

The spouse need not personalize inhibited sexual desire. It is important to maintain your own sexual desire and sexual pleasure. Your sexual interest is a friend and booster for the relationship. If you develop a sexual dysfunction or inhibited sexual desire in response, the problem is further compounded.

SEXUAL DYSFUNCTION AND INHIBITED SEXUAL DESIRE

Which comes first, sexual dysfunction or inhibited sexual desire? This is not the "chicken or egg" argument it might appear. There are couples for whom sexual dysfunction—especially erection problems of men and orgasm problems of women—clearly preceded inhibited sexual desire. Other couples may have had nonsexual stresses such as loss of a job, conflict over child management, illness, or obesity, which lowered sexual desire and subsequently one or both developed sexual dysfunction. Stress from an extramarital affair or major marital disagreement results in severe sexual problems which can include dysfunction and/or inhibited sexual desire. Perhaps the most common pattern is a couple who had a mediocre or unsatisfying sexual relationship and didn't try to improve sexual functioning. Over time, sex became progressively more unsatisfactory with the outcome being inhibited sexual desire. The desire problem robbed the couple of motivation and energy to deal with emotional and sexual issues.

Jill and Robert. Jill was pleased that she hadn't fallen into the traditional female trap of not being aware and interested in sex. As an adolescent, she discovered masturbation and was orgasmic at age fifteen. She enjoyed dating and petting, beginning intercourse at seventeen (this was the norm for Jill's peer group, although she hoped her own daughter would delay intercourse until at least nineteen). Like many women, Jill found it easier to be orgasmic with manual stimulation than intercourse. She enjoyed sexual expression, although she disliked dealing with the roller coaster emotional ups and downs of dating relationships. The worst sexual incident in Jill's adolescence was her contracting chlamydia. However she treated it as a medical issue not a moral one, and there were no long-term physical problems.

At twenty-one Jill expected sex to be a positive and exciting part of her life. She had obtained an associate's degree in office management and was working at a highly respected law firm. Her goal was to be office manager at the firm.

Office affairs are discouraged in all management manuals, but they occur with surprising frequency. Jill was attracted to Robert, who had recently been made a partner—she found him bright and witty. Robert's marriage was coming apart and Jill was there as a friend and emotional supporter. Not surprisingly, intimacy and sexual attraction developed, and their relationship turned into an affair.

Jill enjoyed being with Robert, and found the sexual experiences exciting, but she was put off because he was not open and didn't talk about sex as easily as other men she'd been with. Although he was readily aroused and orgasmic, he was not particularly emotionally or sexually expressive. Jill was orgasmic with Robert, so she was not sure if she was making something out of nothing.

From Robert's perspective, sex was easy and straightforward. He'd begun masturbating at twelve, had his first orgasm with a partner while petting in a car when he was a junior in high school, and first intercourse the summer before he entered college. Sexually, Robert was an automatic and autonomous functioner. In other words, he experienced desire, arousal, and orgasm needing little or no help from his partner. The woman he began dating during his sophomore year in college was the person he married four years later while in law school. Robert was an ambitious, goal-directed person who took the marriage for granted. He found marital sex satisfactory, but erratic in frequency. When under stress he liked "quickie" intercourses to relieve tension.

Robert planned to begin a family after he achieved partner status, and assumed this was what his wife desired. He was shocked to discover that she had an entirely different agenda.

She had been having an affair for over two years and planned to marry this man and move overseas. Throughout the separation and divorce process, she was hostile and cutting in her assessment of Robert. She said he was egotistical, a poor lover, and unaware of the feelings and needs of others. For Robert, Jill was a safe port in a tumultuous storm of attack and negation. Jill respected and liked him, assuaging Robert's self-doubt.

Jill's involvement with Robert was not acceptable to their law firm. She left for a job as assistant office manager in one of the city's biggest law firms. The change was a disaster for her career and a source of resentment in the marriage. A common cause of inhibited sexual desire is resentment over sacrifices made by a woman for a man's career.

Once Robert was assured of Jill's desire to marry, he began to take the relationship for granted. This meant routine and quick sex. Rather than sexual expression improving with time as Jill had hoped, it fell into an unsatisfactory routine. Jill felt committed to Robert so she stifled her feelings of dissatisfaction.

The incident that began the downhill cycle happened on the wedding night. Jill was expecting something romantic and special. Instead, she got the same sex routine. She was furious and they had their worst fight ever. There is a lot to be said for having arguments when you're clothed, sitting up, and not in the bedroom. In bed, especially after sex, there is a vulnerability that is easily elicited with potentially long-term consequences. Robert felt unjustly attacked, which reminded him of feelings from his first marriage. Rather than talking with Jill, he retreated into a protective shell. This was the first and last sexual encounter of the honeymoon. It marked the beginning of Jill's inhibited sexual desire.

Jill regretted losing her temper, but felt Robert's continuing to punish her was unfair. They were at a stalemate. Each felt like a wounded victim waiting for the other to apologize. The longer a stalemate continues, the harder it is to break, and the stronger are feelings of anger and resentment. Anger, more than any other emotion, serves to inhibit sexual desire. The time to deal with desire problems is within six months after they develop. Jill and Robert, like most couples, did not seek professional therapy until sexual difficulties had festered over three years.

The impetus for dealing with the sexual problem was Jill's desire to become pregnant. It is difficult to conceive when you only have intercourse once or twice a month. Robert was reluctant to enter therapy because he was afraid he'd be blamed for the marital, sexual, and fertility problems. Marital therapy is not about blame and refighting old battles. The goal of marital therapy is to revitalize the marital bond and make the relationship satisfying for both partners. After an initial couple session the clinician saw Jill and Robert individually, trying to understand the perceptions and feelings of each.

At the couple feedback session, the clinician emphasized how important it was to make a good faith commitment to revitalize their marital and sexual bond. She noted that it takes most couples at least six months to develop a sexual style that is functional and satisfying. That process had been detoured by the incident on the honeymoon. They needed to work together as an intimate team to communicate, develop comfort, sensuality, and sexual arousal. Most important, they needed to rebuild bridges to sexual desire and be open to the other's touch and sexual requests.

Jill and Robert had a strong desire to maintain their marriage in spite of the sexual disappointments. Jill took her marital commitment seriously, and Robert did not want the stigma of being a "two-time loser." The desire to have a child and the excitement of trying to get pregnant can be a boon to sexual desire.

Although initially hesitant, Robert was willing to devote the time and psychological energy to revitalize marital sex. He found it easy to reawaken his desire and anticipation of being sexual, and took seriously Jill's request to improve the quality of marital sex. Jill found it difficult to build new bridges to sexual desire. She had not expected to be in this situation, and needed to let go of her anger before she could be truly desirous of Robert, Jill was surprised that her ability to be aroused and orgasmic was easier to regain than sexual desire. As positive experiences continued, she developed greater trust in Robert's intentions. The excitement of the impending pregnancy increased Jill's desire.

During the pregnancy, Jill and Robert discussed the importance of maintaining emotional and sexual intimacy. The birth of a first child is a major transition in a couple's life. They were committed to maintaining their hard-won intimacy, and to make becoming a family a positive transition.

PRIMARY INHIBITED SEXUAL DESIRE

Primary inhibited sexual desire is almost always a female problem. It's a direct result of our culture's attempts, directly and indirectly, to stifle female sexual desire until after marriage. Parental and societal admonitions against masturbation and sexual play, warnings about a woman's "reputation," avoiding pregnancy and sexually transmitted disease, and fear of rape, sexual abuse, and being taken advantage of can have a more potent and lasting effect than anticipated. A young woman may not view herself as a sexual person nor value sexual expression. Being married does not magically cure this problem or remove the destructive sexual assumptions. Males do not suffer from primary inhibited desire because they are taught to value sexuality, learn to masturbate to orgasm, and see sexuality as a part of their masculine identity. The same learning opportunities need to be open to women.

Karen. Karen was thirty-two and had been married almost three years. She was a bright, sophisticated woman who was aware of and able to express a number of emotions. However, in discussing her sexual history, it was evident that she suffered from primary inhibited sexual desire.

Karen grew up as a "good girl." She had a warm and close relationship with both parents, and was a more agreeable child than her two older brothers. Both brothers married early, one because of an unplanned pregnancy. Karen's mother encouraged her to attend college and delay marriage. Part of that message was to delay sexuality, which in itself is not problematic.

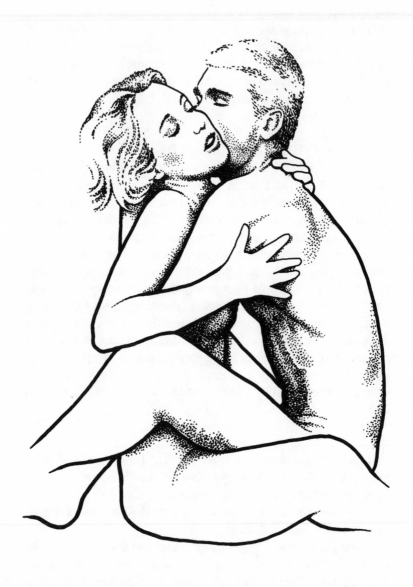

You cannot will or force arousal. Sexual arousal comes from receptivity and responsivity to stimulation.

However, Karen took it to an extreme of avoiding self-exploration and masturbation, dating but staying away from touching except kissing and hand-holding, and remaining as sexually naive and inexperienced as possible. She was socially active in groups and was a "buddy" to several males, but shut out romantic or sexual opportunities. As an adolescent, she came to view her parents' marriage as distant and her mother as a nonsexual woman. She realized they were better at parenting than as a marital couple.

Karen hoped to "fall in love" when she completed college, but that was not to be. She had planned to remain a virgin until marriage. That's much easier to do if you marry at eighteen or even twenty-one, but not realistic if you marry at twenty-nine. Karen naively hoped that marriage and the man would bestow sexual desire on her.

Karen had to increase awareness of herself as a sexual person. Desire resides first in the individual and then is nurtured through the relationship. Karen's ultimate goal was to have an emotionally intimate, sexually satisfying, and secure marriage—a goal shared by most men as well as women. As with other aspects of life, there is a process to go through to reach your goal. "Paying your dues" means learning about yourself, men, relationships, and sexuality. Some of those experiences were positive, but others were difficult and painful.

Karen met Derrick when she was twenty-eight and married him a year later. The sexual relationship with Derrick developed well because Karen had a better understanding of herself and sexuality than at twenty-one. She had learned three major things about sexual desire that would serve her well in the marriage: Sex worked best when 1) her conditions for the relationship were met, (when she felt valued and trusted her partner, and was protected against unwanted pregnancy and sexually transmitted disease), 2) when she was aware of sexual feelings and fantasies and was open and receptive to affectionate and sensual touching, and 3) when her partner viewed her as an attractive, sexual woman and was open to her requests and guidance. As the marriage with Derrick progressed, intimacy and sexuality became more integrated. For Karen as with other women, this is the basis for maintaining sexual desire in marriage.

Inhibited sexual desire (lack of libido) has been considered rare in our sex-oriented culture. However, recent research makes it clear that inhibited sexual desire is the most common sexual dysfunction among couples. People, males especially, are reluctant to admit to desire problems. This is because of our public attitudes toward sex. It's more socially acceptable to have a specific sexual dysfunction than to admit, "I just don't feel like having sex."

Pat and Dan. Pat and Dan regarded marriage therapy as a last resort. Their children were young adults who lived independently. With the house to themselves, they hoped their sex life, which had always been mediocre or worse, would improve.

They labeled the problem as solely Pat's. She had never been desirous of sex, although when they were away on vacation, she would be responsive and orgasmic. Pat's explanation was that with all the other things in her life she did not have the time or energy to be sexually involved. On a vacation, with the pressure off, she was responsive, but in day-to-day life sex was a low priority. She believed she was simply not a very sexual person. It did not bother her that Dan had occasional sexual flings. She did resent his paying a prostitute or spending money on dinner and a hotel room.

Dan felt he had tried everything he could with Pat and that there was nothing more he could do. He told friends he had a "good wife in the house but a dud in the sack" and would lament his lot to women he met, in particular a woman at a massage parlor he frequented weekly. One of the reasons Dan consented to seeing a therapist was the economic argument that it was cheaper (as well as safer) to pay for therapy to improve marital sex than to spend money on dinners, hotels, prostitutes, and massage parlors.

As is usually the case, the causes of Pat's inhibited sexual desire were a combination of sexual and nonsexual issues. Pat felt it was not "right" for her to initiate sex or appear to need sex. When Dan talked about sex, it was with the attitude that "the best sex is dirty sex." Pat wanted no part of that. She could enjoy dirty jokes and was good at telling sex jokes, but could not imagine herself talking about sex comfortably or integrating sexuality into her view of herself as a woman. Dan reinforced this by his traditional double-standard male attitudes.

After two months of therapy, it became evident that Dan's attitudes were a major factor in Pat's inhibition. Dan did not have a high opinion of women. Pat was an excellent mother and homemaker, but these qualities were not valued by her husband. He felt that since he brought home the larger paycheck, he was the most important person in the family. He ridiculed his son for doing woman's work and turning into a sissy because he enjoyed cooking and helped clean the house. Pat had never confronted Dan, but had built up years of resentment. Their marital roles were rigid and stereotyped. This carried into sex: initiation was exclusively Dan's. Sex was to satisfy his needs, and Pat was to be a passive recipient. In sexual and nonsexual ways, Pat's desire was inhibited not only by her attitudes and experiences, but just as strongly by Dan's attitudes and actions.

In order to make a sexual breakthrough, it was necessary for Pat and Dan to focus on the nonsexual aspects of the relationship, especially their rigid view of male-female roles. Anger is a major inhibitor of sexual desire, and Pat, like many women of her generation, expressed anger by turning off sexually. Direct verbal expression of resentment in a nonsexual context is one way of freeing sexual energy. One of the best ways to prevent inhibited sexual desire is to deal with nonsexual issues as they arise, and keep them out of the bedroom. Sexuality is not a good medium to convey nonsexual problems.

At first, Dan was defensive and angry at being confronted with his chauvinism. As the therapist sensitized Dan to the fact that his attitudes subverted their sex life, he began to recognize that they were inappropriate and self-defeating. Pat read about female sexuality and became clearer in identifying the kind of touching and stimulation she would be receptive and responsive to. She did not want to be "worked on" by Dan, who at every moment was evaluating how aroused she was. Pat rebelled against Dan's instruction that she should have one orgasm, which was to occur during intercourse and at the same time as his. In one series of sex therapy exercises the couple refrains from intercourse and engages in a variety of sensual and sexual activities that lead to increased pleasure and arousal. As the therapist had predicted, Dan responded with anxiety and inhibition, whereas Pat was enthusiastic and orgasmic. This made it clear to them that the lack of desire was a couple problem, not solely, or even principally, Pat's. Belatedly, Dan realized that he had a lot to learn about sexuality and relating intimately.

MALE INHIBITED SEXUAL DESIRE

Not only women lack desire and avoid sex. Although it is seldom admitted or discussed, men too suffer from inhibited sexual desire. Approximately 15 percent of males in their middle years report inhibited sexual desire. When couples cease sexual activity, in most cases it is because the man has low sexual desire or is afraid he's lost the ability to function.

Males say they simply lose sexual desire, blaming it on age or the "same old thing with the same old partner." These are easy rationalizations, but are not the real cause. Closer to the truth is that the man has isolated himself from warm, intimate feelings with his wife and takes her and the marriage for granted. He has been drained by the stress of his job, preoccupied by sports, financial, or household interests, and has discounted the importance of marital sex in the middle and later years. He puts little emotional or creative energy into the sexual relationship. Inhibited sexual desire is the self-defeating outcome.

Part of the problem of inhibited sexual desire is caused by lack of awareness; the man does not recognize or accept changes in sexual functioning that come with aging. But because sex is no longer easy and automatic does not mean he has lost desire. He needs to be open to stimulation from his spouse, and to establish comfort and confidence that increased desire and arousal will result. Primary inhibited sexual desire, although it occurs, is relatively rare in males. Young males learn to value sexual expression, engage in masturbation during adolescence, and view sexuality as integral to masculinity. Causes of primary inhibited desire are a paraphiliac (deviant) arousal pattern, conflict regarding sexual orientation, or a sexual fear or secret that alienates him from his partner.

Secondary inhibited sexual desire is as common in males as females. The same knowledge that served a man well in his younger years sabotages his sexuality later on. A male learns sexual desire and functioning in an automatic and autonomous manner. He feels desire, becomes aroused and erect, and experiences orgasm with little or no input from a woman. He views sexual desire and functioning as easy and totally in his control; all the woman needs to do is be there. This attitude sets the stage for him to develop sexual dysfunction and inhibited sexual desire as he ages.

The most frequent cause of secondary inhibited sexual desire is a sexual dysfunction. The most common sexual problem for young males is early ejaculation, also called premature or rapid ejaculation. Often men attempt to deal with this by reducing their arousal and avoiding partner stimulation, which is absolutely the wrong strategy. The focus should be on increasing stimulation and enjoying the give and take of arousal while building awareness and comfort. The most common way for a man to develop erection problems is to engage in "do it yourself" techniques for ejaculatory control, which instead interfere with his arousal and cause him to lose his erectile confidence.

Most males cease being automatic and autonomous performers in their thirties or forties. Since sex is no longer easy and under his control, a man may feel vulnerable and unsure. This serves to reduce sexual comfort and confidence and he is on the slippery slope to sexual dysfunction and inhibited sexual desire. He no longer anticipates being sexual, but worries about performance. Sex is no longer fun and pleasurable, but a task to perform and worry how well he's done. There are increasing periods of sexual avoidance. The old myth that the longer you go without sex, the '"hornier" you get is untrue. The truth is that sexual avoidance feeds on itself. The more irregular the sex, the lower the sexual desire. The male sex hormone, testosterone, increases after a sexual experience. It is regularity, pleasure, and anticipation of sexual expression that builds desire.

No matter how much he wants to, a man with inhibited sexual desire cannot take a magic pill which returns him to automatic and autonomous functioning. He has to develop a new way of thinking about and experiencing sexuality. The key element is to realize that sexual desire and arousal comes *from* the couple interaction, not apart from it. You are responsible for your sexuality, but are no longer an autonomous sexual being. Sexual desire and arousal are tied to what is going on emotionally and physically between the couple. Rather than starting with a spontaneous erection and high levels of arousal, the sexual process comes from touching and stimulation. You need not mourn the loss of easy, autonomous sexuality. You can celebrate the opportunity for more intimate give-and-take sexual expression. Sexual desire comes from positive anticipation and being an active, involved partner in the pleasuring and arousal process.

CLOSING THOUGHTS

Enhancing sexual desire is a couple task. Sexual desire can and does come from diverse sources. Both spouses need to be open to developing and nurturing desire. Relationships in which each person is receptive to nondemand touching both inside and outside the bedroom, where genital touching need not end in intercourse or orgasm, and where the couple share intimately in sexual and nonsexual contexts allows more avenues to experience and express sexuality. The major psychological aphrodisiac is an involved and aroused partner. Your desire and arousal facilitates your spouse's desire and arousal.

Inhibited sexual desire is the most complex and common sexual dysfunction. If it lasts more than six months, we suggest you seek professional therapy because desire problems become more severe and chronic. The sense of frustration, blaming, and avoidance builds.

You deserve to feel good about yourself as a sexual person. Sexuality can play an integral role in energizing the marital bond. Sexual desire is not magic; it can be nurtured and enhanced.

13
DEALING WITH AROUSAL PROBLEMS

Sexual functioning is arbitrarily divided into four phases: desire, arousal, orgasm, and emotional satisfaction. This chapter will focus on issues and problems with arousal, the second phase. Almost all the focus has been on the male's erection, and amazingly little attention has been paid to female arousal. There has been an inordinate emphasis on medical interventions to enhance erections. Although these can be helpful and appropriate for many couples, they are often misused and overused in a desperate effort to build and maintain erections.

The key element in sexual arousal is receptivity and responsivity to stimulation. Positive anticipation and sexual desire facilitates, but is not necessary for, arousal. Arousal is easier for people who are regularly orgasmic, although individuals who have difficulty with orgasm can and do enjoy being aroused. Couples who are emotionally satisfied with their marriage report easier arousal, although sexual arousal can occur even when there is severe relationship dissatisfaction.

Ideally, arousal would be part of a natural progression starting with a sense of emotional connectedness, leading to sexual desire, which flows into receptivity and responsivity, leading to high levels of arousal, naturally culminating in orgasm, followed by a sense of emotional satisfaction. Not every sexual scenario can or should follow this format, which is an unrealistic expectation—and anything that predictable would be boring. An arousal problem is best conceptualized and treated as a couple problem. Arousal needs to be understood in the context of the couple's entire pattern of emotional and sexual relating.

Lack of arousal, manifested by lubrication problems in the woman and erectile problems in the man, is more distressing than orgasmic problems. The spouse feels sexually inadequate. Lack of sexual pleasure and arousal can cause doubts as to whether there is love and attraction and if the marriage is viable. It is often the more basic issues—lack of communication, anger, unresolved relationship problems, extramarital affairs, in-law problems, individual problems that impinge on the marriage and lack of time together—that block sexual receptivity and arousal. Some couples have a strong and viable bond, but poor sex undermines the marriage. Although relationship problems can cause sexual problems, the converse is also true. Sexual problems can cause individual and marital problems, especially low self-esteem and emotional alienation.

Arnold and Faith. One factor that encouraged Arnold and Faith to marry was their excellent sex life. Arnold had divorced his first wife after three years and had been single two years before meeting Faith, who was five years younger than he. This was Faith's first marriage. After eight years of marriage and two children, their sex life was a bitter disappointment. It was difficult to pinpoint when things began to degenerate, but the period after the birth of their first child was particularly problematic. Faith felt the burden of taking care of the baby was entirely on her. She was enraged when she discovered that Arnold was involved in an extramarital affair that had begun early in her pregnancy. This revelation, combined with the fatigue Faith felt because taking care of the baby disrupted her sleep, caused her to be less sexually responsive (this is a common pattern for new mothers). When she was not well lubricated, intercourse and, especially, entry was painful. Faith suggested using a lubricant, such as K-Y jelly, but Arnold

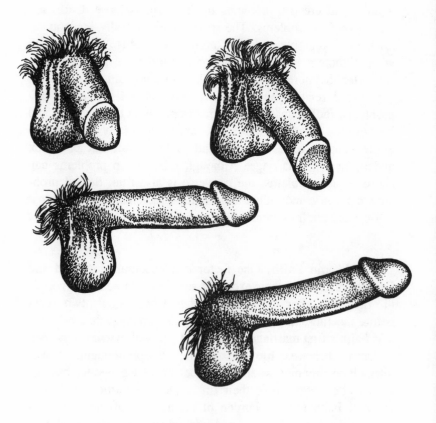

Erections can and do wax and wane. Understanding and comfort with that process is key to regaining erectile confidence.

became irrationally angry at that idea. In trying to force insertion when she was poorly lubricated, Arnold had trouble maintaining his erection. As he worried about the state of his erection
and fell into the pattern of being a sexual spectator, his arousal
waned and so did his erection. Although sex went well on
occasion, with increasing frequency Arnold was not able to
maintain or, at times, even obtain an erection. When they did
proceed to intercourse, Faith found it uncomfortable and unsatisfying since Arnold was rushing to be sure it would work.

One night there was a destructive blow-up. Faith was aroused,
but Arnold felt a great deal of performance anxiety and was
unable to get an erection. Faith lashed out at him, partly because she felt humiliated and rejected. She accused him of no
longer loving her and obtaining all his sexual satisfaction through
affairs. In fact, Arnold had experienced erectile difficulties in
his one affair. However, his pride had been hurt, so rather than
admit to sexual difficulties, he claimed that sex was great in
affairs which proved she was a castrating bitch. This caused
Faith to doubt her femininity and attractiveness, and she responded by counterattacking and striking out. Their argument
was a vivid example of violating the guideline to avoid sexual
discussions in bed after a bad experience. Hurtful memories and
decreased feelings of trust dominated their relationship.

The next three years were punctuated with fights and short-
lived attempts to get the sexual relationship back on track.
Having a second child was an effort to shore up the marriage.
Arnold at thirty-nine and Faith at thirty-four were seriously
considering divorce. However, they still cared for each other
and their children. They decided to attend a group program on
sexual dysfunction.

The initial focus was on replacing sexual performance demands with a series of nondemand pleasuring exercises. For the
first two weeks, there was a ban on intercourse. Faith and
Arnold found, with the pressure for performance gone, that they
were able to respond to touching with pleasure and arousal.
After an experience during which Arnold was aware that, in a
forty-five minute period, his erection waxed and waned four
times, they had a frank conversation about sexual feelings and

the state of sex in their marriage. Arnold was feeling more secure about his ability to regain an erection. Waxing and waning is a natural physiological function, not a sexual problem. A key element in regaining erectile confidence is developing an awareness of, and comfort with, the waxing and waning process, and realizing that the erection will wax again if not blocked by performance anxiety and taking the spectator role. Sexual arousal occurs when both partners are receptive and responsive to sexual stimulation.

Arnold told Faith that he not only found her attractive, but that her sexual interest and responsivity was the most important factor in his arousal. Arnold revealed that he was more functional with Faith than during his affair. This latter self-disclosure was particularly difficult because it made him more vulnerable. He realized that, despite all the hurt and pain they had experienced, Faith continued to love him, and he clearly loved her. Faith said that for her to feel more responsive sexually she needed Arnold's active involvement in caring for the children so she could have time to think of herself as a sexual person and spouse, not just a mother. Arnold's involvement with child care and household tasks was a concrete demonstration that he valued the marriage.

Faith needed Arnold's commitment to sexual fidelity. With a greater feeling of trust, his attention to the cares and chores of their life, and a renewed commitment to the marriage, Faith gave herself permission to become involved sexually and let go of her resentments and inhibitions. Her arousal, lubrication, and orgasmic response returned. Faith found that multiple stimulation both before and during intercourse was the key to her sexual satisfaction. Arnold was aware that he didn't always need a firm erection to satisfy Faith and with that realization his anticipatory performance anxiety dramatically lessened.

DEALING WITH AROUSAL PROBLEMS

Couples need to trust each other and the relationship enough to go through the somewhat clinical and sometimes tedious techniques necessary to overcome an arousal dysfunction. Sexual relearning is not necessarily romantic or passionate. You need to establish a comfortable touching relationship, and then move to more pleasurable and sensuous forms of stimulation. Genital stimulation and multiple stimulation results in greater excitement which naturally culminates in orgasm. Although it sounds easy and straightforward, it requires a great deal of emotional involvement and couple time and effort. You need to deal with frustration when things don't go well. Stay with the cycle of practice and feedback until you feel more comfortable and satisfied with your couple sexual style. Sexual arousal is much more than a series of techniques and exercises; it is an expression of your emotional and sexual intimacy. Be aware of positive expressions of sexuality in marriage, not just genital arousal and intercourse.

Sexual techniques that facilitate arousal are best thought of as the one-two punch. One is nondemand pleasuring, and two is multiple stimulation. Receptivity to affectionate and sensual stimulation, followed by responsivity to genital, erotic stimulation, leads to sexual arousal. You cannot force vaginal lubrication nor can you will an erection. Sexual arousal is a natural physiological response to effective sexual stimulation. The naturalness of sexual response is illustrated during the sleep cycle. While sleeping restfully with no interfering thoughts, a woman will go through two to five cycles of vaginal lubrication and a man will experience two to five cycles of waxing and waning of erections. Sexual arousal is natural for both women and men.

What interferes with arousal? The major factor is self-defeating expectation caused by our old nemesis the male-female double standard. A second factor is a specific fear or inhibition that blocks arousal. The third, and usually easiest to overcome, involves the couple not having developed sexual scenarios and techniques that build arousal. The three following cases illustrate each block.

Delores and Nathan. Delores and Nathan had been a couple sixteen years and had been married for eight. They were in their late thirties and had two children under five. Nathan was always

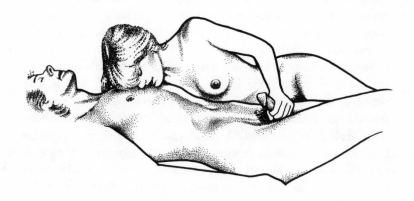

Your partner is your sexual friend—be open to her touch and stimulation.

the sexual initiator. He would stimulate Delores to get her sexually interested and aroused. Nathan had spontaneous erections and needed no stimulation from Delores. She was used to the passive role and being given to and Nathan enjoyed the active, seducer role. The expectation was that Nathan would be ready and willing for sex any time Delores was.

The male-female double standard might work for couples in their twenties, but causes trouble when couples reach their thirties; few couples in their forties find it usable. As they age, men and women become more alike sexually. This can result in better quality sex if it is understood and accepted. Expectations built by the male-female double standard have to change dramatically. At its best, sexuality is mutual sharing, a cooperative giving and receiving of sexual pleasure. When a man no longer functions automatically and autonomously he has to be open to her stimulation. The woman can initiate, be sexually active, and enjoy a range of sexual expression instead of being stuck in the passive role.

Delores found this an easier transition than Nathan. She genuinely enjoyed initiating sex play and showing sexual interest. It was intriguing to realize that she could excite him with her hands and tongue. Arousing Nathan was arousing for Delores. Nathan came to understand that an involved, aroused partner is a major sexual aphrodisiac. However, he still felt uncomfortable that he needed Delores's stimulation to obtain and maintain arousal and erection.

Nathan was used to intercourse on his first erection. Discovering that erections waxed and waned was new. Delores enjoyed the process of helping him, but Nathan longed for the days of easy, predictable sex. Quality sex is involving and interactive. When a man reduces his defensiveness and inhibitions, it is arousing for him too. Nathan still preferred to go to intercourse on his first erection, but was more accepting of other sexual scenarios. He came to understand that interactive sex was satisfying and creative, although more variable.

Sarah and Sam. Much of the time the major roadblock to sexual arousal involves a relationship issue. Sarah and Sam met while married to other people. Sarah had married seven years before because of a pregnancy and had a seven-year-old daughter; her husband wanted them to stay together for the daughter's sake. Sarah realized that they were better as parents than as spouses or lovers (they had not had sex in three years). Sarah's parents had stayed together "for the sake of the children" and she did not want to repeat that pattern in her life.

Sarah saw her relationship with Sam as a transition to being single again. She was attracted to Sam and enamored by his attention and passionate wooing of her. Six weeks after meeting Sam, Sarah left her husband. Up to that point their sex had been excellent. They met at hotels for "nooners" and had gone away for a weekend. Sarah remembers it as the most sexually free time of her life.

During his marriage, Sam had adopted a pattern of affairs that lasted from two weeks to two years. After eight years of marriage, he had developed erection problems with his wife. Although they occasionally had intercourse, he never regained his erectile confidence with her. Erections were easy early in a new affair, so he told himself his arousal problems reflected the fact that he was a man who required new partners. Sam preached to his friends, "Man is not meant to be monogamous." When erection problems began, he immediately dropped the relationship.

Sarah told Sam that the coming months were likely to be a "crazy time" for her. Her first priority was to get her life back to an equilibrium and set up a co-parenting arrangement. Their relationship would not be as much fun or as sexual and she would understand if he left. Sam surprised himself by staying with Sarah. He rationalized that even if the sex wasn't as frequent it was still passionate and fulfilling. Sarah's arousal remained high—sex with Sam was a tension-reducer and energized her to cope with problems. She was finding it difficult and draining to convince her husband to stop fighting to get her back and to accept the inevitability of the divorce.

Sam's first problem with erection occurred four months after Sarah's separation. He was sure Sarah hadn't noticed, but he rushed intromission and ejaculation so that he wouldn't have an erectile "failure." Sam was sensitized and self-conscious about his erection, and tried to downplay and avoid sex. About two months later, they were being sexual at Sarah's initiation and Sam lost his erection right before intromission. Sarah was a sexually aware and sophisticated woman who knew this occasionally happened with men and didn't make an issue of it. Sam felt humiliated, turned his bad feelings on Sarah, and blamed her aggressiveness. Sarah felt unjustly attacked and they got into the kind of destructive fight couples have about sexual issues. Sarah fully expected Sam to terminate the relationship, which was Sam's intent in provoking the fight. He found to his amazement that he couldn't do it. Sam had come to love and respect Sarah, and couldn't walk away from the healthiest intimate relationship he'd ever had.

The next two years were an emotional roller coaster for them. Sam separated from his wife and Sarah decided to live with him to see if they were a viable couple. Could Sarah and Sam sustain their commitment and establish an intimate and secure second marriage? Sarah realized that being angry with Sam and feeling emotionally distant squelched her sexual desire. When she was receptive to sexual touching, she had little difficulty becoming sexually aroused. As she became aware of this and communicated it to Sam, their sexual relationship progressed. Sam understood that the exact same sexual scenario which would result in passionate feelings and multiorgasmic response when Sarah was open resulted in dead feelings when she was not desirous.

Sarah did not take Sam's erectile difficulties personally nor did she view erection as a sign of his love or her sexual attractiveness. She correctly labeled the erectile difficulty a "psychological block." Too much of a man's self-esteem lies in his penis. This was certainly true for Sam. The key to regaining sexual comfort and confidence is viewing your partner as your sexual friend, seeing sexuality as pleasure giving and pleasure receiving rather than a pass-fail performance, and viewing intercourse as part of the pleasuring process. Sam heard these concepts in therapy sessions, read them in sexuality books, and experienced with Sarah the waxing and waning of erections. Sarah stimulated him manually and orally, and guided his penis into her.

As is true of many males, Sam was stubborn when it came to changing sexual attitudes and behavior. The emotional break-through came one morning when he awoke with an erection. He tried to initiate a quick intercourse, but lost his erection. Rather than allow him to slip into a feeling-sorry-for-himself mood, Sarah asked to cuddle. She was responsive to his touch. When he began to stimulate her toward orgasm, she moved his hand from her genitals to her chest and said she just wanted to feel good and be close. Touching continued for ten minutes and Sam found himself receptive to her touch and realized he was becoming erect. He did not focus on his penis, but stayed with feelings of emotional closeness and pleasure. In the next twenty minutes his erection waxed and waned two or three times, but he was not particularly concerned. When Sarah got on top and guided him into her it seemed the most natural thing possible. After that experience, sex between Sarah and Sam went smoothly with no major roadblocks. On those occasions when he was not aroused and his erection was not firm, they felt free to engage in alternate sensual and sexual scenarios.

Tara and Juan. When a sex therapist encounters a couple whose major problem is lack of knowledge and awareness of sexual technique, she can almost guarantee a successful out-come. Tara and Juan were in their mid-twenties, married two years, and feeling desperate about their sexual life. Each felt loving and desired to be sexual. Both were able to be orgasmic during masturbation. However, each time they had intercourse Juan would ejaculate early and Tara was neither aroused nor orgasmic. Juan was so discouraged by his ejaculatory dysfunction that he avoided sex. They viewed the problem as Tara's not having an orgasm, with the cause being Juan's early ejaculation.

After an assessment including individual sex histories, the therapist reconceptualized the problem as an arousal dysfunc-tion. Tara was not aroused before beginning intercourse. Juan was so concerned with early ejaculation that he avoided Tara's touch. Juan was bewildered, but willing, when the therapist suggested that he spend more time pleasuring Tara, and be open to Tara's touching him, including genital stimulation.

The first step in arousal is being receptive to sensual, nongenital touch. Like many young men with early ejaculation, Juan's touch was rapid, rough, focused on the woman's genitals, and goal-oriented toward intercourse. He needed to learn to touch in a slow, nondemanding, pleasure-oriented manner. He was surprised and pleased when Tara responded to his touch. Tara told Juan she would feel more aroused if he were open to her touch. Juan was not comfortable lying back and being passive, but he did enjoy being touched while he caressed her. Slowing down the sexual scenario was pleasurable for Tara. She knew she could respond sexually, but the rapid, goal-oriented sexual scenario Juan had used dampened her arousal. As Juan become comfortable receiving genital stimulation, his ejaculatory control gradually increased. The key to learning ejaculatory control is building comfort, not reducing arousal. Tara found, as is true of many women, that if she were aroused and/or orgasmic during the pleasuring phase, it was easier to be aroused and orgasmic with intercourse.

AROUSAL ISSUES FOR WOMEN

Although the media focus since the 1960s has been on female orgasm, women knew that wasn't the real problem. When she experienced sexual desire and arousal, orgasm was a natural culmination of the sexual process.

The traditional answer to female arousal problems was to label the woman "frigid." Happily, that term has fallen into disrepute in the professional community and is decreasing in popularity among the lay public. The new "sophisticated" answer is to blame the man: "He's a lousy lover." The old trap was to blame the woman; the new trap is to blame the man. Blaming is easy, but does not facilitate sexual arousal.

As with other sexual problems, arousal is best conceptualized as a couple issue. The focus is on the woman communicating and working with her partner to enhance comfort, receptivity, and responsivity. She takes an active, involved role in the pleasuring process. The key element is to communicate and guide her spouse, either by putting her hand over his or making verbal requests. The male is not the sexual expert nor can he read her mind. What he can do is be open to her requests and guidance. She needs to increase sexual awareness and take responsibility for her arousal.

Although some women prefer to be passive while being stimulated, most women prefer the "pleasuring" concept. Pleasuring involves giving and receiving sensual and sexual touching that is nondemanding and non-goal-oriented. Involvement, comfort, pleasure, and arousal are steps in the process of sexual expression. The more involved the woman, the greater the arousal. The man performing "foreplay," i.e., servicing the woman to get her ready for intercourse, is unacceptable. Both attitudinally and in terms of technique there is a world of difference between "servicing" and "giving" to a partner. Pleasuring involves a genuine giving and receiving of sensual and sexual stimulation. The major sexual aphrodisiac is an involved, aroused partner.

The sexual scenario usually culminates in intercourse. However, intercourse is not the sole, or even primary, goal of the pleasuring process. A major mistake couples make is to initiate intercourse on the man's timetable, which means when the woman has begun to vaginally lubricate. Why proceed to intromission then? We suggest that couples initiate intercourse on the woman's timetable and that she guide intromission. Continue with pleasuring until the woman is feeling moderately aroused rather than beginning intercourse early in the arousal cycle.

A woman is the expert on her vagina; let her guide intromission. This allows the man to receive additional penile stimulation as well as reduces the possibility of discomfort or pain on intromission. Some women are subjectively aroused, but lubricate minimally. In this case, she might consider routine use of a vaginal lubricant at the beginning of the pleasuring period. Some women prefer K-Y jelly because it is a sterile lubricant, others find it too clinical. We suggest using a lubricant that has a pleasant smell and feel, and is hypoallergenic so it will not cause vaginal irritation.

Intercourse has traditionally been viewed as the man's domain. The woman's role was to be the recipient. If she moved more and had orgasm during intercourse, all the better. In truth, intercourse is as much for a woman as a man. Whether a woman is orgasmic during intercourse is not the major factor in satisfaction. She can be an involved, aroused partner during intercourse whether she's nonorgasmic, orgasmic during the pleasuring period, orgasmic during intercourse, or orgasmic during afterplay. There are a number of techniques that can facilitate her pleasure and arousal during intercourse. These include her controlling coital thrusting, using intercourse positions that allow more freedom of movement (woman-on-top or lateral-coital), engaging in multiple stimulation during intercourse, and/or using simultaneous clitoral stimulation. Clitoral stimulation can be done by either the woman or the man. Sex does not end with the man's ejaculation; her sexual needs and arousal are equally important. This includes requesting manual stimulation during afterplay. Female arousal is integral to a couple's sexual relationship.

ISSUES IN MALE AROUSAL

Arousal problems in males have received an inordinate amount of attention in the past few years. A woman doesn't need to be aroused to engage in intercourse, but a man does. The male views his erection as a "union card," without which he is not a man. "Real sex" is reduced to his penis, intercourse, and ejaculating intravaginally. This obsessive focus on erection and intercourse has not served the male or the couple well. Sexuality is based on pleasure. When viewed as performance, it inhibits intimacy and sexual expression. Males needs to view sexuality more broadly as a range of feelings, sensations, and scenarios.

What is the reality of male arousal and erection? Most males, though certainly not all, learn about erections as automatic and autonomous. Adolescents make jokes about spontaneous erections at awkward times. Sometime in their mid-twenties to mid-thirties, these easy automatic erections decrease in frequency, and by the mid-forties have basically disappeared. Although men would rather talk about anything other than erection problems, the reality is that by age forty, over 90 percent have had at least one experience when they haven't been able to obtain or maintain an erection sufficient for intercourse. Thus, we find that the most feared male sexual problem is almost a universal occurrence.

Why do men have occasional erection problems? The potential causes are almost too numerous to mention. They include too much alcohol, stress about a nonsexual issue such as work, money, or a sick child, interruption by the telephone ringing or a knock on the door, angry feelings, side effects of medication, the partner being uninterested or demanding, not feeling sexual but believing it's not masculine to say no, not receiving enough stimulation, a vascular or neurological problem, rushing into intercourse, trying too hard to please your partner, fatigue or stress, using a "do-it-yourself" technique for ejaculatory control but reducing arousal instead, feeling distracted and not sexually interested. In other words, a myriad of physical, psychological, relational, situational, and sexual factors can interfere with arousal and erection. The penis is not an automatic-function machine; it is influenced by numerous feelings and factors. Occasional erectile problems are a normal part of male sexuality and cannot be prevented. There is no reason to fear or overreact to occasional erection difficulties.

In one-third of males, the erection problem lasts at least a month. For approximately 10-15 percent the erection problem becomes chronic. This means that over twelve million males have erectile dysfunction. The problem is most prevalent for males over fifty, but can affect men in their teens and twenties. What is the most common cause of erectile dysfunction? Performance anxiety. When sexuality is taken out of the context of pleasure and viewed as performance, a man is halfway to developing sexual dysfunction. He becomes stuck in the syndrome of negative anticipation-unsuccessful experience-sexual avoidance. A large percentage of males with erectile insecurity develop inhibited sexual desire. Interestingly, when couples stop being sexual, over 95 percent of the time it is the man who stops the sexual activity. The major reason is erectile dysfunction, which causes desire problems, and eventually he gives up in frustration. "Use it or lose it" is true; the more sex is avoided, the harder it is to retain sexual functioning.

What is the best way for a man to deal with an erection problem? Think of it as a couple issue and avoid falling into the trap of guilt, blame, and diminished sense of masculinity. The key is to gradually regain your comfort and confidence with arousal and erections. The therapeutic process includes instituting a temporary prohibition on intercourse, to reduce performance anxiety and provide an opportunity to reinvolve yourself in the pleasuring process. Sexuality is an active process of giving and receiving pleasure. Sex is not a spectator sport. When you are a passive spectator on the state of your penis you remove yourself from the arousal process. An important awareness is that your erection can wax and wane and wax again. Until you have at least two good erections with nonintercourse sex, do not attempt intercourse. Intercourse is part of the pleasuring process, not a pass-fail sexual performance test.

We suggest that the couple seek professional sex therapy to deal with erectile dysfunction since it is easy to get frustrated and lose motivation. A sex therapist is in a position to help you decide whether there is a need to undergo specialized assessment of neurological, vascular, and hormonal factors. There has been a dramatic increase in medical interventions, especially surgery to insert a penile prosthesis (an irreversible procedure) and injections to increase blood flow to the penis. Although these can be of great value to couples when the male has a chronic medical condition that makes erection impossible, they can be inappropriate technological attempts to deal with a psychological or relationship problem. Males find medical interventions appealing because the responsibility is taken from them and a return offered to automatic and autonomous erections. Before utilizing a medical intervention, especially one which is irreversible, we strongly suggest that the couple consult a urologist and/or sex therapist together and discuss the implications for their emotional and sexual life.

CLOSING THOUGHTS

Arousal is an integral element in the process of desire, arousal, orgasm, and emotional satisfaction. An arousal problem is best viewed as a couple issue. We suggest seeking professional therapy rather than trying to deal with the problem by yourselves, especially if it has lasted more than six months. Identifying blocks—whether psychological, relational, or sexual—and increasing receptivity and responsivity to sexual pleasure are the key elements in resolving arousal problems.

14
LEARNING TO BE ORGASMIC

In the 1960s, orgasm was treated as the centerpiece of human sexuality. Orgasm and sexual satisfaction were thought to be synonymous. Orgasm is a positive and integral component of sexuality for both women and men, but orgasm is *not* the most important part. The essence of sexuality is giving and receiving pleasurable touching. Orgasm is the natural result of sexual awareness and comfort, receptivity and responsivity to stimulation, multiple stimulation leading to high levels of arousal, and letting go as the culmination of sexual pleasure.

Men and women learn about sexuality and orgasm in different ways. Not surprisingly, their problems with orgasm are different. The most frequent male problem is early ejaculation and the most typical female problem is low frequency of orgasmic response. There are physiological reasons for this difference, but the most relevant causes are differences in self-awareness and sexual technique.

The great majority of males learn to be orgasmic via masturbation. By age eighteen, over 90 percent have masturbated to orgasm. Although women masturbate, they do so in fewer numbers than men. Rates of female masturbation increase with age and marriage. Women who are orgasmic during masturbation find it easier to be orgasmic in couple sex. Many readers find this concept bewildering. In prior generations, masturbation was blamed for a variety of psychological and sexual problems. The empirical evidence is clear: body self-awareness and masturbation facilitate orgasm in partner sex for both women and men. In fact, the treatment of choice for preorgasmic women (those who have never been orgasmic by any means) are female sexuality groups which emphasize self-exploration and masturbation. Success rates are over 85 percent. Once aware of your individual sexual response pattern, it is easier to transfer that learning to partner sex. We are not saying masturbation is the best way to learn to be orgasmic, but it is the easiest and most direct way.

Some males suffer from ejaculatory inhibition, also called ejaculatory incompetence or retarded ejaculation. It is extremely rare for a male to be unable to ejaculate under any circumstances. More common is the male who can ejaculate by means of masturbation and partner manual or oral stimulation, but does not reach orgasm during intercourse. As males age, about 15 percent develop intermittent ejaculatory inhibition, which means they do not reach orgasm even when aroused and desirous of being orgasmic.

EARLY EJACULATION

The most common orgasmic problem for males is early ejaculation, also called premature ejaculation, rapid ejaculation, or involuntary ejaculation. The majority of males begin their sexual lives as early ejaculators. Perhaps 50 percent of males under twenty-five have a pattern of early ejaculation, and it is a complaint for about one-third of adult couples. There are four reasons for couples to work together to develop ejaculatory control: (1) enjoying the full range of sexual sensations improves the quality of the sexual experience for both the man and the couple, (2) early ejaculation is a major percursor to other sexual dysfunctions, especially erectile problems when the man decides to use "do it yourself" techniques to lower sexual arousal, (3) early ejaculation interferes with female sexual response and can be a major source of misunderstanding and

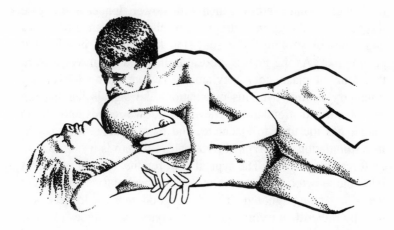

You cannot will or force an orgasm, it is a natural response to heightened sexual arousal and psychologically letting go.

conflict in the couple's relationship, and (4) when the man develops comfort and pleasure, and reduces anxiety and performance-orientation, these learnings serve to inoculate him against sexual problems that occur with aging. It is better to learn this in your twenties and thirties, before a crisis, than to deal with a more severe dysfunction.

The key in ejaculatory control is to maintain arousal and replace anxiety with comfort. Learning ejaculatory control is a gradual process. The couple practices the "start-stop" technique, first with nonintercourse stimulation, then with intercourse in the woman-on-top position and minimal movement (the quiet vagina exercise), then with slower, longer intercourse thrusting. Gradually they progress to other intercourse positions and types of stroking. The start-stop technique is just what it sounds like. As the male's arousal builds and he moves toward the point of ejaculatory inevitability (where he no longer has voluntary control over his ejaculation), he signals her to stop movement and stimulation. They wait a few seconds until he no longer has the urge to ejaculate, and then resume slow, rhythmic stimulation. The typical trap males fall into is trying to rush or force the process. The typical trap for the woman is to feel intercourse is too mechanical and/or that her sexual feelings and needs are being ignored. There are good reasons to seek sex therapy rather than trying ejaculatory control techniques on your own. The techniques are powerful and helpful, but couples need to maintain motivation, emotionally support each other, and continue to practice and progress if they are to comfortably integrate ejaculatory control into their lovemaking.

FEMALE ORGASM

The most common complaint couples have is that the woman does not reach orgasm during intercourse. More husbands than wives complain about this. The myth is that a woman should have an orgasm just like a man, i.e., a single orgasm occurring during intercourse. Female orgasmic response is more complex and variable—notice, we don't mean better or worse—than male orgasm. The woman might be nonorgasmic, singly orgasmic, or multiorgasmic. Orgasm can occur during the pleasuring period, during intercourse, or in afterplay. There are books and magazine articles touting six kinds of orgasms, extended orgasms, G-spot orgasms, vaginal orgasms. All this makes for great talk show and bar talk, but scientifically it's nonsense. There is not a meaningful difference between orgasms through intercourse or nonintercourse sex (the famous vaginal versus clitoral controversy). An orgasm is an orgasm whether from masturbation, cunnilingus, vibrator stimulation, intercourse, or manual stimulation. Each woman has her own pattern(s) of orgasmic response. If the woman is regularly orgasmic during partner sex then there is not an orgasmic dysfunction—it's as clear as that.

Among adult woman, approximately 10 percent have never been orgasmic by any means. An additional 10 percent are regularly orgasmic with masturbation or vibrator stimulation, but not during partner sex. Of the 80 percent of women who are orgasmic during partner sex about 65 percent have been orgasmic during intercourse. This means that a substantial proportion of orgasmic women are never orgasmic during intercourse. To label them as dysfunctional is ludicrous. If the woman enjoys intercourse and is regularly orgasmic during partner sex, she and her spouse should celebrate instead of worrying that there's something missing.

Among women who can be orgasmic during intercourse, the majority find it easier to reach orgasm with nonintercourse stimulation. There is not a "right" or "normal" pattern for all women. The important thing is to develop one or more patterns that are comfortable and satisfying for you. Women who are multiorgasmic are more likely to experience that through cunnilingus and/or manual stimulation than intercourse. Another pattern is to be orgasmic during pleasuring, making it easier to be orgasmic during intercourse. Contrary to popular myth, women who are multiorgasmic do not report four or twenty times more pleasure than women who are singly orgasmic. Nor do women who are orgasmic during intercourse report greater satisfaction than women who are orgasmic through nonintercourse sexual expression.

Some women have a strong preference to be orgasmic during intercourse. Many couples utilize simultaneous clitoral stimulation during intercourse, others do not. When it comes to female orgasm, "let a thousand flowers bloom" is descriptive of the variety of satisfying sexual expressions.

CHANGING FEMALE ORGASMIC RESPONSE

There are treatment strategies and techniques to help women develop satisfying orgasmic patterns. Female orgasmic problems are also best conceptualized as couple problems and treated with the help of a professional sex therapist. Preconditions for the resolution of an orgasmic problem are to establish an intimate, open, communicative, trusting relationship, develop comfort with nondemand pleasuring, and engage in multiple stimulation. The woman needs to be aware and take responsibility for her sexuality. You cannot will or force an orgasm, it is a natural response to heightened sexual arousal and psychologically letting go. Very few women experience initial orgasm during intercourse. Masturbation is the most common means followed by partner manual or oral stimulation. Vibrator stimulation is also helpful in achieving an initial orgasmic experience.

Female orgasm is one of the most widely written about and discussed aspects of human sexuality. Increased awareness that a woman has a right to expect orgasm as a natural part of sexual expression is positive. The conflicting negative trend is that female orgasm has become "The Big O," an unrealistic performance demand for the "right" kind of orgasm each time. Instead of increasing awareness and comfort, this burdens female sexuality with the same performance orientation that has proven so harmful for male sexuality. The healthy association is between sexuality and pleasure. When women, or men, think of orgasm as a performance goal they are halfway to developing sexual dysfunction. Orgasm is a natural, integral part of being a woman. Orgasm is a result of self-awareness, sexual self-acceptance, receptivity and responsivity to effective stimulation, and the ability to let go and experience climax. Orgasm is *not* a measure of female sexuality, a performance goal, nor a means of proving something to yourself or your spouse. Orgasm is part of the pleasure-giving and pleasuring-sharing process, not something apart from it.

A major factor is that the sexual scenario move at the woman's pace, not the man's. He must be open to her requests and sexual guidance. The pleasuring process is a gradual transition from nongenital to genital stimulation, but not until she is desirous and receptive. If the woman is not open to breast, vulva, or clitoral stimulation this is counterproductive and detracts from the arousal process. Most women prefer indirect to direct clitoral stimulation, and that it proceed in a slow, tender, rhythmic manner. As arousal builds, the woman needs to stay with her own rhythm of touching and movement and not switch to the man's.

The bridge from moderate levels of arousal to orgasmic response is multiple stimulation. Multiple stimulation includes maintaining rhythmic stimulation around the clitoral area while adding additional stimulation such as manual or oral breast stimulation, stimulation of the mons and/or anal area, kissing and caressing, intravaginal finger stimulation, vibrator stimulation, and/or rubbing the penis against her breast or vulva. Some women prefer to be passive and accept stimulation, but most prefer more active involvement, giving and receiving stimulation. Examples include touching and stimulating the man, engaging in sexual fantasy, moving her body in a rhythmic manner, giving and receiving oral stimulation simultaneously, and/or being in a standing or kneeling position which allows greater freedom of movement.

Letting go and being orgasmic involves psychological, sexual, and relational factors. Psychologically, the crucial factor is letting go of the sense of control. Trust yourself and your spouse and don't be self-conscious about being aroused and orgasmic in front of him. Orgasm is an intense, erotic experience that lasts only a few seconds. You deserve to be orgasmic; give yourself permission to experience the pleasures of orgasm.

The major sexual factor is use of "orgasm triggers." These techniques allow you to heighten arousal to the point of orgasm. Orgasm triggers vary from woman to woman. They include tightening leg and/or thigh muscles, which builds tension until it bursts forth in orgasm, giving yourself to a sexual fantasy and letting it culminate in orgasm, asking your partner to stroke faster and harder as you go toward orgasm, and/or verbalizing that you're "going to come." Sexual stimulation is focused, erotic, and rhythmic. As you reach high levels of arousal, use orgasm triggers to help you let go and feel the satisfaction of orgasm.

Relationally, there is a caring and trusting bond. It is not up to the man to work his magic and give you an orgasm. Arousal and orgasm are your responsibility. His role is being an involved, giving, caring partner, open to your guidance and requests. There are a number of relational factors that interfere with orgasm, especially feelings of alienation or anger. Orgasm is natural to an intimate sexual experience and reinforces the couple bond.

Lily and Robert. It is not unusual for both partners to have difficulty with orgasm. One of the most common problem situations includes a man who is an early ejaculator and a woman who is nonorgasmic during intercourse. This was the situation for Lily and Robert, a couple in their early thirties who had been married four years. Robert had always been an early ejaculator, but this had not bothered him. He thought of sex as intercourse, and saw himself as a lusty, passionate male. Lily had been orgasmic, although infrequently, with other partners. She enjoyed Robert's sexual passion, but became disillusioned even before they were married.

Robert was very intercourse-oriented and spent less than five minutes on foreplay, which was mechanical and perfunctory. He was erect and ready to go before his clothes were off. It wasn't just his ejaculation that was rapid, it was the whole approach to sex. Like males who have spontaneous erection and early ejaculation, Robert did not want to be touched because he mistakenly believed it would speed his ejaculation. Lily saw him as a selfish sex partner, uninterested in her sexual feelings and needs. He was worried because Lily wasn't involved or interested in sex. His reaction was to be more intense and intercourse-focused which only compounded the problem.

Robert and Lily made the classic couple mistake. After intercourse, she expressed her frustration, which caught him off guard and his defensiveness quickly became offensive. They had a half-hour yelling and crying match, blaming, calling names, and "hitting below the belt." Robert called Lily "frigid" and a sexual neuter. Lily called Robert a "pig" and the worst lover she'd ever had. You are very vulnerable when you're nude and lying in bed. It is the wrong time to voice frustration or sexual complaints. It's easy for this to get out of control, as it did for Lily and Robert, and degenerate into a "pissing contest." The only good thing that came out of the debacle was a decision to seek therapy rather than to allow the marriage to degenerate.

The key concept in sex therapy is to view the dysfunction as a couple problem and avoid the guilt-blame cycle. The issue is not blame—arguing whether your partner caused or didn't cause the problem. The key point is that both must work together to develop a couple sexual style that is comfortable, functional, and satisfying. As Barry says during therapy, "Sex is a team sport—you support your mate, you don't turn on her."

Lily and Robert felt relieved that they were addressing sexual concerns in a constructive way. In conducting individual histories, it became apparent that Robert had shifted from being unaware to feeling that the whole burden was on him, especially to make sure that Lily had an orgasm during intercourse. Changing from one extreme stance to another is not helpful. Robert mistakenly believed it was his responsibility to make Lily respond just like him, to have a single orgasm during intercourse. To accomplish this all he thought he needed to do was prolong intercourse for ten minutes. The therapist explained to Robert that this was a self-defeating way to view ejaculatory control. Sex was not a performance he gave to win Lily's orgasm. Robert was to learn ejaculatory control for himself, to increase his awareness and comfort and enjoy a range of pleasurable sensations, especially being inside Lily and engaging in slower, longer thrusting. Robert was primarily responsible for ejaculatory control, and needed Lily's active involvement.

Lily was responsible for increasing her awareness and orgasmic response, and would need Robert's active involvement. Lily's sexual pattern had been to follow the man's direction. Her premarital partners had been like Robert, very intercourse-oriented. She'd had two partners who spent time attending to her needs and tried to arouse her. One used a variety of stimulation positions and Lily remembered being aroused and orgasmic on occasion. However, as soon as he felt she was sufficiently aroused he moved to intercourse. The other man was insecure about erections, and preferred manual and oral stimulation. He was the partner with whom Lily had the most orgasms, but she tired of working so hard to get him aroused and was put off by his avoidance of intercourse.

Lily liked Robert's enthusiasm for intercourse, but missed manual and oral stimulation. She had been too embarrassed to make those requests. Lily had to be active and aware, to take responsibility for her arousal and orgasm, and give up the fantasy that all she needed was his ejaculatory control.

The couple feedback session was particularly helpful in giving Lily and Robert an understanding of the problem and a way to approach it as a cooperative, intimate team. Especially important was the concept that each person needed to assume prime responsibility for his or her sexual awareness and then share with, support, and encourage the spouse. Robert did not initially see the value of starting with nongenital pleasuring, but after the first three exercises he was a convert. The idea of slowing down and enjoying pleasuring was important, but of special value was his openness to receiving stimulation. For Lily, taking initiatives, especially developing pleasuring scenarios and guiding Robert in what was arousing for her, was of special value.

One serendipitous effect of sex therapy is that some women learn a multiorgasmic response pattern. Lily was excited to find that she could develop sexual scenarios and positions which were arousing for her. She enjoyed Robert combining oral breast stimulation with manual clitoral stimulation, while she rhythmically moved her pelvis. She particularly enjoyed a pleasuring position where she was standing and he kneeling, touching her breasts and vulva. She found that switching intercourse positions greatly increased her arousal, particularly when there was multiple stimulation throughout. Lily was pleased to discover that when she was involved and creative, orgasm was relatively easy.

Robert found sex therapy more difficult than Lily. This is not unusual, women are more open and receptive to sex therapy strategies and techniques than men. Lily blossomed under the permission-giving context of the sexual exercises. Robert was learning and experiencing new things, but was distracted by worries about sexual performance. He found it difficult to let go and fully enjoy the pleasuring process. When they began the manual start-stop ejaculatory exercises, Robert became noticeably tenser. The therapist wisely suggested they desist from those exercises for two weeks, and that Robert engage in masturbatory exercises aimed at identifying the point of ejaculatory inevitability, and practice the start-stop procedures on his own. Once Robert successfully mastered the ejaculatory control process via masturbation, he was more confident and motivated for couple exercises. It was hard for him to be in a position where he needed help from Lily. But that is the heart of sexual intimacy, seeing your spouse as your intimate friend and being open to sexual requests and guidance.

Intercourse was reintroduced as part of the pleasuring process via the quiet vagina exercise. This entailed Lily guiding intromission from the woman-on-top position, with minimal movement. The experiences of having Robert inside her for ten minutes and feeling the sensations of intravaginal containment was good for Lily, but not erotic. Robert realizing that he could be in the vagina that long was very reinforcing. Learning ejaculatory control is a gradual process. It involves experimenting with different types and rhythms of thrusting and intercourse positions. Not surprisingly, Robert found it hardest to maintain ejaculatory control when he was on top and doing short, rapid thrusting. His control improved in other intercourse positions and he enjoyed slower, more pleasure-oriented sexual processes, variations on the side-by-side position and stroking that was longer and at various speeds. He eventually learned to slow down thrusting rather than stopping altogether.

Lily found that her orgasmic response was similar to that of many women: it was easier to be orgasmic with manual and oral stimulation. When she was orgasmic during intercourse, the sensations were not noticeably different. Both Lily and Robert valued the experiences of her being orgasmic during intercourse, but did not make it a performance criterion. More important, orgasm and intercourse were an integral part of their lovemaking. The most enduring lesson of the sex therapy was the importance of staying with the pleasuring concepts and being an intimate team.

Jack and Trudi. The problem of intermittent ejaculatory inhibition increases in the middle years. As many as 15 percent of couples experience this. Jack was an early ejaculator in his mid-twenties; it was not until the mid-thirties that he developed ejaculatory control. He became more comfortable with sex and open to Trudi's stimulation, and their intercourse frequency was two to three times a week (a regular rhythm of intercourse promotes ejaculatory control). Trudi did not begin having orgasms until two years into the marriage, but by her mid-thirties was orgasmic in over two-thirds of their sexual experiences. Trudi found arousal and orgasm easy. Her favorite sexual scenario was to be active in kissing and caressing which allowed her to be open to Jack's stimulation. Trudi especially enjoyed receiving a sexual massage which integrated non-genital and genital touching. As arousal built, Trudi moved toward orgasm by thrusting her pelvis while Jack was stimulating her with his penis, hand, or tongue. Jack enjoyed her arousal, which added to his own.

Throughout the book we have made the point that you cannot rest on your sexual laurels. This is the trap that Trudi and Jack fell into. By their late forties, Jack had begun to feel that sex was easier and better for Trudi than for him. He never voiced his feelings, which festered and grew more invasive. It is normal for a male occasionally not to reach orgasm, the major reason being that his arousal is moderate and remains so throughout intercourse, so that he doesn't reach a peak toward orgasm. The male is considered to have a problem of ejaculatory inhibition when during at least one in four opportunities he is aroused and desirous of having a climax but is unable to. Over the previous five years the occurrences of ejaculatory inhibition had increased, but neither Jack nor Trudi addressed the problem. Orgasm does not exist in a vacuum. Trudi's arousal and orgasm also began to decline. Their sexual relationship was on a downhill slope and the next stop was likely to be inhibited sexual desire.

Trudi took the initiative to break the cycle. She bought *Male Sexual Awareness* and underlined three concepts she thought were particularly relevant—multiple stimulation, requests for special sexual scenarios, and using orgasm triggers. She left this under Jack's pillow with a cute note about winning a sexual prize. She also bought a pair of sexy short pajamas that provided a nice touch.

What turned things around was a sexual scenario in which Trudi brought Jack to orgasm orally, something they hadn't done in five years. The next morning she told Jack that she really enjoyed helping him to get excited and have an orgasm, that it was arousing for her when he was aroused. Jack acknowledged how nice it had been and how free he felt. He shared a story about a work colleague who had been frustrated and resentful toward his wife, had acted out by having an affair with a divorced, younger secretary, and how this had disrupted the work environment and his marriage. Jack told Trudi that he valued their life and marriage, but admitted that he'd been frustrated with their sex. He didn't expect miracle changes, he said, but last night had been a great start.

Jack read the book, and identified the problem: as Trudi became more aroused she'd stopped stimulating him, and his level of arousal became inhibited. He'd never said anything because he felt he was being a crybaby, but he needed her continued stimulation for his arousal to build to orgasm. They agreed to experiment and play together to develop more interactive and exciting sexual scenarios. Middle-years sex is not as easy and predictable for a man as youthful sex. But if he can make sexual requests and enjoy the give and take stimulation, middle-years sex can be higher quality and more satisfying. An involved, aroused partner really is the major sexual aphrodisiac.

CLOSING THOUGHTS

Orgasm is not what sex is ultimately about. The essence of sexuality is giving and receiving pleasurable touching. Orgasm is a natural, positive, integral part of pleasure-oriented sexual expression for both women and men. Orgasm occurs as a natural progression of the pleasuring process, not as a performance goal apart from it. Each spouse is responsible for her or his orgasm. Being orgasmic is part of the intimate couple sexual experience.

15

EFFECTS OF ROLES AND RESPONSIBILITIES ON SEXUALITY

A neighbor remarked after reading initial drafts of this manuscript that it sounded great, but didn't describe marriages she was familiar with. "Typical psychologist," she said, "talking about the way things should be, not the way they really are."

Consumers have legitimate complaints about self-help marriage and sex books. The guidelines are too glib, the people in the case studies too self-sufficient, things turn out perfectly, and people have their cake and eat it too. Self-help books err in the direction of being Pollyanna-ish, promising that if you follow their easy 1-2-3 rules you can have a perfect life, marriage and sex. But couples themselves err in expecting too little intimacy and sexual satisfaction in their marriage.

It is possible to fulfill your roles and responsibilities while enjoying a sexually satisfying marriage. You don't need to choose between being a responsible parent, employee, and church member and being a sexually happy person. These life components can and should complement each other. Research evidence demonstrates that happily married people enjoy and do better in their careers than those with poor marital and/or family situations.

221

Married couples, especially those in their thirties, forties, and fifties, feel burdened by responsibilities. Society depends on middle-years people to be productive as well as care for younger and older generations. Financially, the middle years are the most lucrative, and middle-years people have the most power and influence in the culture. The trade-off is that they have the most responsibilities—to their children, the community, jobs, homes, and elderly parents. You have a multitude of roles and life is much more complex and demanding than when you were a child or young adult.

Couples who view their roles and responsibilities as burdens, either as restraints to be shucked off in becoming liberated or as unending pressures that must be carried through for the good of the family and society but to the detriment of themselves, fall into the trap of feeling resentful and blaming. The result is decreased marital and sexual satisfaction. You can view roles and responsibilities as creative challenges that at times are burdensome and energy draining but, on the whole, enhance the meaning and quality of your life. This attitude facilitates marital and sexual satisfaction. You needn't make yes or no choices between the joys of pleasure-oriented sexuality and your responsibilities within the family, such as attention to parenting, being a conscientious breadwinner, religious practice, and being a home-oriented person. Your personal, family, marital, and sexual life will be enhanced if you integrate sexuality into your marriage and see roles and responsibilities as integral to the marriage. Congruence among attitudes, behavior, and feelings enhances psychological well-being and marital satisfaction.

Regarding the relationship between sexuality and religion, couples who have positive, nonrepressive, nonguilt-oriented religious beliefs enjoy better marriages and marital sex. It has been erroneously reported that the more religious a person is, the less sexually happy he is. Recent data indicates just the opposite. Moderately religious people report greater marital and sexual satisfaction than nonreligious couples.

Erica and Don. Erica and Don were involved with a church-sponsored couples' reading and discussion group. A prime focus was how their lives and responsibilities had changed in sixteen years of marriage.

Erica had dropped out of college, left home, and was working in a furniture store when she met Don. Don was from a conservative background and had returned to his parents' home after completing college. His goal was to save money and open his own business. At thirty-eight he was the owner of a successful sporting goods store. Erica had stayed home with their children, now thirteen and ten, until they'd begun school. Then she returned to college, finished her degree, obtained a master's, and recently had been promoted to physical therapy supervisor. With two children, two careers, two cars, and a mortgage, Don and Erica had a busy and full life.

Nevertheless they were worried about their life direction. Did the way they lived reflect their values or were they simply stumbling along day to day? At the birth of their first child, they had resumed church attendance. Their church group read about and discussed issues of values and life meaning. Sexually, they had always been a functional couple, but in the past few years there had been a subtle decrease in the spontaneity and pleasure of their lovemaking. Like so many couples in the middle years, when they talked about sex they did not talk about their own sexuality, but concerns about adolescent sexuality and political arguments about sexual attitudes and behavior in America.

They read books on spirituality, life meaning, and the role of sex and marriage. Some of the ideas such as going to pornographic movies struck them as immoral. Others, like sanctioned extramarital affairs and open sharing of details seemed unrealistic. And still others—weekends away at resorts, for example—were just not appealing. Concepts that focused on marital enhancement, especially the use of multiple stimulation during lovemaking and permission to enjoy couple time without feeling guilty, were incorporated into their lives. It really is okay to leave business calls unreturned for an hour, okay not to volunteer for another community *ad hoc* committee, and okay not to be the parent who drives all the kids to every Saturday soccer game. To Erica and Don, spirituality meant having a sense of inner peace and a family and religious connectedness. They set aside time after church on Sunday to play tennis with another couple and then go to brunch.

Like other middle-years couples, Don and Erica had "a lot of balls in the air." As is true for many couples, it was the "sexual ball" that was the easiest to drop. Erica was interested in their sexual experiences being more intimate, especially incorporating nondemand pleasuring techniques. For that to happen she had to take a break from the frenzied pace of the day. She needed time by herself to relax before being with Don. High on Erica's list of priorities was attending to the needs of their children—she was distressed by the number of "latch-key children" in the neighborhood. This meant paying attention to the children's physical needs and getting them from place to place, but more importantly listening to them, being genuinely interested in their activities and projects, and knowing the children's friends. How could these conflicting needs for attention to children and needs for individual and couple time be met?

On nights when Don and Erica planned to get together sexually, Erica would spend time with the children before and during dinner. After dinner she would read, sew, or take a relaxing bath. Don took charge of homework, activities, and getting the kids ready for bed. Instead of waiting until late to start a sexual interaction, Don met Erica in the bedroom about ten, and began by talking and caressing instead of immediately starting sexual stimulation. This was pleasuring time, not goal-oriented foreplay. Their talks and looks served as psychological seduction which, combined with nondemand pleasuring, restored a sense of interest and anticipation to couple sexuality.

At church and in the discussion group, people talked of marriage as a sacrament. An intimate marriage and loving family was conceptualized as a religious vocation. Intellectually, that sounded good, but what about sex within marriage? These ideas were particularly difficult for Don. He enjoyed receiving oral sex because it was daring and exciting. When Erica talked about how much she enjoyed receiving oral sex, Don had uneasy, hard to articulate feelings. He felt that getting so much pleasure from an act that was not described in the Bible and did not involve the union of man and woman seemed sinful. Although intellectually Don accepted the "God as love" view and objected to religion's traditional role of inhibiting expression of pleasure because it was sinful, it was not easy for him to integrate sexual feelings and practices with religious beliefs. Feelings do not change just because attitudes change or you try something new; it was an ongoing process. Emotional openness, and sharing experiences, feelings, and perceptions resulted in a positive integration of sexuality and spirituality in Don and Erica's marriage.

ROLES AND RESPONSIBILITIES

In the stereotype of the traditional family, the roles of men and women are clearly spelled out and *very* separate. The males's roles are instrumental: bring home money, discipline children, do home repairs, be the family head. The woman's roles are nurturing: provide emotional caring for children, cook and clean so your husband can relax, service him sexually, maintain a loving family, and be sure everyone's—except your own—emotional and practical needs are taken care of.

In our marriage, we try to discard these cultural stereotypes. We strive to make our marital roles shared and equitable. Each of us has skills and interests, so we don't split things fifty-fifty. The "liberated" concept of everything being shared equally is unrealistic and rigid. We emphasize equity in power and task distribution rather than fifty-fifty equality in all aspects of life. Flexible does not mean chaotic. For a family to operate, there has to be structure and role assignments; each person has to take responsibility for significant tasks. Shared roles and responsibilities means being willing to negotiate and reach agreements. Be aware of your interests and competencies and use them as a basis for the roles you choose instead of obeying sterotypically masculine or feminine role prescriptions. Each person has to be open and flexible, even the best thought out system has glitches. Humor is the best antidote to power struggles and frustrations.

Sometimes tasks involve a reversal of traditional roles. An

example is that Emily is mechanically skilled and takes prime responsibility for household repairs, whereas Barry enjoys doing dishes and is responsible for kitchen clean-up. Discipline of the children is shared, as is active involvement in caring for and nuturing them. Providing a parental model of flexibly sharing tasks is an excellent way for children to learn about adult roles of women and men.

Money is a major issue in almost all marriages, and can be especially stressful at certain times. No matter how much you have, it never seems enough for all your desires and responsibilities. In the worst of situations, the man complains that his only function is to "bring home the bacon," and berates his wife for spending money. The woman may feel emotionally abandoned by her spouse, who seems to value his job over his marriage and family, and takes satisfaction from accumulating material goods—at the same time indirectly getting back at the husband who does not satisfy her companionship and affectionate needs. This is an extreme situation, yet too many couples fall into this trap. Money issues are among the most disruptive in marriage.

Guidelines for sexual communication are relevant when communicating about financial matters. Each couple will have their own money-management style, depending on background, habits, and values. You will manage better if you view money decisions as a couple issue with joint responsibility. When you are honest with yourselves and each other about how much money is earned, and where and for what it is spent, and make requests for how money is allocated, financial issues can be dealt with in a productive manner.

One definite "no-no" is a trade-off between money and sex (we're not talking about sex for pay). Don't fall into the trap of saying "If we have sex this special way, I'll buy you a winter coat," or of being angry about a money issue and refusing to have sex until you get your way. Marriages in which money and sex are used as bargaining points run a high risk of developing emotional and sexual problems. You play a money power game where no one wins and the marital bond is the ultimate loser.

The three issues that engender the most emotional tension in marriage are sex, children, and money. Couples talk about sex with a therapist much more readily than they reveal their financial affairs. Handling money responsibly in a marriage is a difficult task. Couples who set up a successful money management system have a real marital strength.

PARENTING

Having and parenting children is a major role and responsibility. That is why we emphasize the importance of planned, wanted children. Your roles and responsibilities change dramatically according to the age of the child. The stresses and joys of parenting a baby are quite different from those you'll experience with a toddler, which in turn are quite different with a preschooler. When you send your child to school you may feel relief from the constant responsibilities, but are faced with new ones—interact with teachers, school officials, community athletic teams, music or dance instructors, coordinating play activities with other parents. Couples hope that as children become older they will require less time and energy, but that's not true. Parenting does change in terms of skills and attitudes, but at every stage being a parent is a time-consuming and challenging task. Even during the golden years of childhood, ages seven to eleven, children want and need guidance, support, and time from parents.

Parenting an adolescent can be as draining as parenting a baby except that you have more control over babies. A favorite metaphor of ours is the "emotional bank account" theory of parenting. You establish positive bonds with a baby and young child and gradually accumulate a wealth of small deposits in the parent-child emotional bank account. In adolescence, there are few deposits and often many withdrawls, some of them massive. You want to be sure there is a positive balance left.

We believe theoretically and personally that parenting is one of life's major challenges and sources of satisfaction. Parenting goes better when the mother and father share roles and responsibilities in an equitable manner. Men can learn to change diapers and be there to give emotional support. Women can be disciplinarians and coach sports teams. Talk about and agree on a style of parenting that fits your interest, skills, and life circumstances. Remember, each child is unique. Because a parenting approach worked well with one child doesn't mean it will fit the needs of another.

Parents need to be aware that they are individual people and a married couple with a need for time and privacy to be sexual. Balancing individual, couple, and parental roles is a complex challenge, but worthwhile for all involved. The husband-wife bond is the most important one in the family. If that is functional and satisfying, other family relationships will thrive. In the long run, putting aside time to be an intimate couple facilitates being better parents.

COMMUNICATION ACROSS GENERATIONS

Especially concerning sexual issues, one of the most difficult positions is the middle one, between your parents and children. You don't want to be the sexual morality arbitrator. Grandparents may warn parents that they are being too liberal with their children, that sexually kids and society are "going to the dogs." Sexual communication and understanding is rare between middle-years couples and their parents. This problem is even more severe if the aging parents have had a poor sexual relationship or a spouse has died.

The solution is simply to refuse to be the middleman. Encourage grandchildren and grandparents to talk directly with each other. They probably will not agree, but this communication allows your children to gain a different perspective on the world. They'll get to know their grandparents as people who possess a wealth of experience and can provide an historical and cultural background, that also includes the issue of sex and marriage. Children will learn that grandparents can adapt and change. Exposure to children and adolescents can have great value to grandparents. The child's desire for knowledge and new outlooks provides a challenging and broadening experience for grandparents. The role of the grandparent is downplayed in contemporary America, but it can be of great value to you and your children.

Your role with both older and younger generations is to provide caring, support, and guidance, and not to feel entirely responsible for them (this last is especially important in regard to aging parents and young adult children). The line between being involved and caring, and feeling overly responsible is difficult to maintain. Some couples begin by being authoritarian and domineering, and then overreact and become overly permissive and ineffectual. Either way, you don't meet the needs of grandparents or children. A healthier approach is to care, support, and help deal with transitions without falling into the trap of being altogether responsible and imposing your will.

Nowhere is the caring, responsible approach more crucial, yet more difficult, than in the area of sexual awareness. In the "good old days," there was a widely believed myth that there was *one* right way to achieve happiness and it was the parents' responsibility to teach children that right way. Parents were judged to be successes or failures by whether their child was successfully married. It was a shock to a parent when five, ten, or twenty years later a married child went through a divorce. Was it the parent who failed? Should the parent revert, feel responsible, and assume a burden of guilt for the "failure"? There are three myths imbedded in this attitude:

1. There is only one right way to be happy.
2. Parents are primarily, or even entirely, responsible for the successes or failures of their adult children's marital and sexual lives.
3. A divorce is always a sign of failure.

A more rational attitude is that your responsibility as a parent is to love, educate, guide, listen to, and support your children. It is inappropriate and self-defeating to evaluate yourself as a person or parent by how well your children are doing at a given point in time. As they become young adults, they assume responsibility for making decisions about their lives, including decisions about relationships and sexual expression. It is not helpful to them or you to feel guilty about the past. You will be in a better position to help in the present transition or crisis if you don't feel burdened by guilt and regrets from the past.

Nick and Sally. Nick and Sally had a difficult time organizing their lives. This was a second marriage for both. Sally had first married at seventeen, had two children, divorced at twenty-three, raised the children alone for nine years, and married Nick at thirty-two. Nick's first marriage was initiated at nineteen when the woman he'd been dating became pregnant. After fourteen years of a bad marriage, a drinking problem, major career shake-ups, and two more children, Nick and his wife had the sense to realize that this was not a viable marriage. Four years later, Nick married Sally. Sally's daughters lived with them; Nick's children visited weekends and summers and during difficult periods would stay longer.

As individuals, Nick and Sally had to get their lives together. This included finding better paying and more satisfying jobs. Even more important, they had to develope a stable and intimate marital bond. Added to this were the stresses of parenting children and stepchildren. "Blended" families are different from nuclear families. They are more exciting and challenging, but also more complex and stressful. "The most important relationship is our marital bond," was written out and displayed over Nick and Sally's nightstand. Remembering this got them through some rough times. They knew that if they could make their marriage good and keep it good, other things had a better chance of working out. This strategy had a positive effect on the entire family.

The relationships and strains in blended families are more complex and require awareness of emotional boundaries between family members. They also require more tolerance and acceptance of different patterns of thinking and behaving. Babies and young children required much time and attention and Nick and Sally were glad to be done with those responsibilities. There is even more stress in parenting adolescent children because you are dealing with the transition to greater independence. One adolescent had an unwanted pregnancy she chose to terminate and an adult child was divorced after two stormy years of marriage.

Nick and Sally decided that the best thing they could do was to give guidance and support when asked, and provide a model to demonstrate that adults grow and change. They had a strong commitment to nuturing their marital bond. They were upset by family problems, but tried not to feel guilty or overly responsible for their adult children's lives. They were consistent in their caring and support, willing to listen and give advice when asked, but unwilling to take over for their children. In the long run, this strategy was successful both for their marriage and relationships with their adult children.

A recurring fantasy for many couples, including ourselves, is that if only we didn't have so many responsibilities and so many roles to play, everything would be perfect. If only we lived on a Caribbean island! Like most "if only" thinking, this gets you nowhere—not to mention that there are a multitude of marital and sexual problems on Caribbean islands.

Make an honest and frank appraisal of your life and how you handle roles and responsibilities. Have you allowed jobs, community projects, or unproductive time—watching soap operas, gossiping on the phone—to dominate your life and interfere with your marriage? If so, you need to reorder your couple and family priorities. What is usually needed is less of a total life change and more setting aside time for yourselves as people and an intimate couple. Some couples need to confront a major issue (for example drinking, being controlled by the job, depression and alienation, anger at a parent or child, overspending credit cards, filling your life with activities so you don't deal with your spouse) and resolve to make a major life change. We suggest consulting a therapist rather than trying to do this on your own.

CLOSING THOUGHTS

This chapter is not meant to be Pollyanna-ish: we are not saying that you can meet all your sexual, personal, couple, family, career, religious, and community needs with never a compromise. You have to assess honestly how you organize your life and your roles and responsibilities, set priorities, make hard decisions, and stick by your agreements. Even the best of couples have to negotiate difficult issues and accept imperfect agreements. What should not be compromised is couple time and sexual satisfaction. Treating yourself well and taking time to be a sexually intimate couple allows you to handle roles and responsibilities instead of seeing them as a burden to be resented. Sexual expression is good for you as a person and for your marital bond. It energizes you to deal more effectively with your roles and responsibilities and facilitates a better quality of life. Feeling good about your marriage and sexuality will pay long-term dividends for your parenting and job.

16

A COST-BENEFIT ANALYSIS OF
EXTRAMARITAL AFFAIRS

Many couples will read the title of this chapter and decide to skip it. They would rather not think about or discuss, much less deal with, the issue of extramarital affairs. The reality is that an extramarital affair by one or both spouses occurs in almost two-thirds of marriages. It is an almost universal experience for both women and men to fantasize about extramarital relationships and have the opportunity to engage in one. Even former President Carter admitted to lustful thoughts about other women. This chapter is not for just a small minority of errant spouses; the issued raised affect the great majority of couples.

No matter what you read in pop psychology books or hear on talk shows, extramarital sex is not a black-and-white issue. The meaning and impact of an extramarital affair must be understood in the context of the marriage. An affair could be a strategy for leaving a poor marriage or be an impulsive one-shot fling; it might serve as a way of preserving a marriage in which sex is nonexistent or be a means of expressing anger; it may be an expression of an individual need or a way of gaining the approval of the "boys" during an out-of-town convention, a way to get back at a spouse, a means of trying to make up for past failures, or a way to bring romance and excitement into an otherwise dreary existence. Each affair has its reasons, its set of characteristics, and its consequences to the individual and marital bond.

We will not engage in abstract arguments about the rights or wrongs of extramarital sex. We will discuss marriages in which affairs occurred and explore how couples dealt with them. We present guidelines for preventing extramarital affairs for couples who wish to go that route as well as guidelines to deal with discovered affairs in order to minimize their impact.

DEALING WITH AFFAIRS

The popular ideas of "open marriage" and "honestly communicating all details and feelings" are, in our opinion, inappropriate and destructive. Although the concept of open marriage was greeted with intellectual excitement and, for a time, became chic, empirical evidence strongly indicates that it is not a functional model for marriage or extramarital affairs. An extramarital affair entered into to fulfill your needs might best be dealt with by not sharing it with your spouse. Revealing feelings and details is not being open and honest, but is a means of expressing hostility or of ridding yourself of guilt. It serves to get feelings off your chest and to burden your spouse with doubt, questions about sexual inadequacy, and a need to do something about the affair. Ask yourself why you are "telling all" and whether your spouse really wants to know all. If you have thought out your motivations, and sense that your spouse does want to know, then by all means share all; but discuss the affair with a constructive purpose, not with a vindictive "let me tell you who it was, exactly how we did it, and how many orgasms we had" manner.

One danger in not informing your spouse is that she may find out in an embarrassing or traumatic manner and will feel humiliated. If the affair was motivated by a problem in the marriage, the spouse is still in the dark about your dissatisfaction. It makes more sense to confront the dissatisfaction directly rather than to express it indirectly through an affair.

Whether the affair is ongoing or has been terminated is crucial. It is easier to talk about and deal with an affair that is no longer active. At some level of awareness, most spouses *do* know about an affair, although at first they may react with hurt surprise and insist that they never suspected. On closer examination, it usually becomes evident that there were clues and dissatisfactions that the spouse tried to ignore and discount. Even the children are usually aware that something has been going on in their parents' lives.

TYPES OF AFFAIRS

Extramarital relationships are very complex; be aware of this complexity when thinking about your affair or your spouse's. Very arbitrarily, you can divide affairs into three categories:

1. High opportunity-low involvement affair, characterized by impulsiveness, little emotional connection, and often paid for (massage parlor, prostitute). This is the most common type of male affair.
2. An ongoing affair, a continuous relationship largely sexual as opposed to emotionally based, enjoyable but not committed, and not a direct threat to the marriage.
3. The comparison affair, characterized by this relationship meeting significant sexual and/or emotional needs not met by the marriage. This could be a one-year, ongoing love affair or a highly charged three-week relationship. People leave their marriages for comparison affairs. This is the most common type of female affair.

The male/female double standard has a great deal of influence on how people react to affairs. The traditional double standard holds that males can play around as long as they don't get the woman pregnant, contract a sexually transmitted disease, or fall in love, but that the woman *must* remain faithful. Extramarital affairs somewhat follow this pattern—approximately 50-60 percent of men have an affair sometime during their marriages, most of which are high opportunity and considered by them to be of minimal importance. Approximately 25-40 percent of women have affairs, which tend to last longer and are more emotionally involving. On two grounds, wives' affairs have more impact on the marriage:

1. They diverge from the double standard and are more threatening and distressing to the spouse.
2. A comparison affair is a more serious threat to the marriage.

HOW TO DEAL WITH AN AFFAIR

Each person will have different feelings, values, and experiences regarding an extramarital affair. If the marriage is to be viable, the revealed affair must be dealt with. Dealing with it can mean anything from having one emotional fight and then letting it go to entering marriage therapy and discussing feelings of hurt, anger, vulnerability and trust for a year or longer. Typically, dealing with the affair involves a series of emotional interactions—tears, anger, threats—and then more rational discussions of the affair and its meanings. The couple discusses the causes of and feelings about the affair and comes to an explicit agreement regarding future extramarital relationships.

A helpful guideline is to focus not on the affair but on the marriage. Dealing with a revealed affair means discussing dissatisfactions with the marriage and concrete plans to make the marital bond stronger. It does not mean continually going over details of the affair. One way of considering an affair is as a cry for help from a marriage that is not faring well. If the message is attended to and the crisis dealt with, the marital bond can become stronger. Certainly there are more direct and less stressful ways to convey the message of a need for marital or sexual help. However, if an affair has occurred, it does little good to blame, induce guilt, wallow in self-righteousness, or engage in "if only" thinking. If you want to revitalize your marital relationship, focus communication in the present and future and on your marital bond.

This guideline is particularly relevant if the affair remains unknown to the spouse. If you are going to try to revitalize your marriage, the crucial first step is to end the affair. This is more complex and considerably harder than it initially sounds. Affairs are easier to get into than out of. You have to free yourself from the affair in order to have the time and emotional energy to focus on the marital bond.

It is true that when there is an extramarital affair it is more likely that a marriage will end in divorce. It is not true that extramarital affairs are the chief cause of divorce. Typically, the problems that precipitated the affair—sex, money, individual dissatisfaction, child-rearing issues—are what cause the relationship to disintegrate, not the affair itself. Affairs are harmful for marriages, but they are not the major cause of marital dissolution.

Some people use an affair as a way of getting out of a poor marriage and/or as a transition to being single again. There are marriages that cannot recover from an extramarital affair. If respect and trust cannot be restored, trying to "save" the marriage is a hopeless task.

Doreen and Al. Doreen and Al were in their late forties. Four years before, their marriage, already in a stressful phase, had been badly shaken by the revelation of Doreen's affair. Al's small business was in decline and the money from Doreen's job, which had gone toward house furnishings and vacations, was now needed for ongoing expenses. Doreen was resentful that Al didn't ask for or acknowledge her financial help during this period. He also denied that he was depressed, avoided talking about problems, drank heavily, stayed out late, and had a brief sexual fling. Doreen was being sexually ignored, and suspected that Al was having a number of affairs. He was paying little attention to the children, which put another burden on Doreen. Previously, when Al had been depressed, drinking, and staying away from the family, she had accepted his behavior passively. This time her resentment peaked, and she rebelled against being at his beck and call.

Doreen was happy to receive the attentions of a buyer at work, and within three weeks had embarked on a passionate affair. Doreen loved the attention, as well as the idea of a younger man finding her sexually attractive. They went to nice restaurants and had sex at fashionable hotels. Al was so self-involved that he didn't notice how often Doreen was gone or that the kids' needs were not being met. This situation continued for five months. It was twelve-year-old Gordy's being arrested for shoplifting that brought the issue to a head. Al ranted and raved, demanding to know why Doreen didn't supervise the children and where she had been. Doreen said she wasn't putting up with him any more and was leaving, at which time a very ugly scene ensued, with name-calling, pushing, and threats.

Doreen found the lover relationship easier when it was an affair and not a substitute for marriage. The affair began to sour after she left Al. The young man did not want to deal with her feelings of confusion, anger, and guilt. On his own, Al was feeling even worse. His business, marriage, and children were all going to hell, and he felt lonely and unable to cope. Although many people would have sought therapy at this time (and before the crisis would have been even more appropriate), Al and Doreen were stubborn enough to keep the situation in its uncomfortable holding pattern for another two months.

It was Al who made the first move toward reconciliation. He sold his business, began working in a temporary job, and felt a strong need to get his life together; for him that meant reestablishing the security of marriage and family. He resented Doreen's having an affair, but very much wanted her back. Doreen did not enjoy being separated, but was reluctant to reenter a marriage in which there were financial problems, resentment, and Al's history of depression, noncommunication, and heavy drinking. Yet it was difficult to turn her back on eighteen years of marriage and to reject Al's request to give their marriage a good-faith effort.

Before returning to living together, they had emotional and serious conversations about their marriage and affairs. Doreen refused to take the role of the "bad guy," although she did regret, and apologized for, her affair. They realized that Al's business problems had caused marital conflict. They made an agreement not to have sexual affairs, and to recommit to marital fidelity. This is the most common agreement for those who are trying to rebuild their marital trust bond. Al agreed to talk things over when he was upset instead of ignoring Doreen and drinking to excess. When business was difficult he would exercise and use other stress reduction techniques. He committed himself to abstaining from alcohol when there was work-related stress.

Four years later, their life was on more solid ground, partly because they were doing better financially and working at jobs they liked. They valued their marriage and sexual life and devoted time and attention to it. Successfully dealing with the crisis had made them feel better about themselves as people, and strengthened their marital bond. They felt better prepared to be parents of adolescent children, which can put stress on the most stable marriage.

Anger, guilt, confusion, and distrust are emotions that people typically attach to extramarital affairs. Envy, a sense of reawakening, heightened sexual desire, and an appreciation of spontaneity are also possible outcomes. Couples whose sex lives have been mediocre or almost nonexistent for years report a sexual reawakening after an affair. Instead of taking the marital partner for granted and being satisfied with the same old marital sex, there is renewed sexual desire. Their sexual life can be more creative and satisfying.

Joe and Gail. Joe and Gail were thought to be the perfect couple. They liked and respected each other, enjoyed doubles tennis and giving dinner parties, were involved parents and enjoyed their children, supported each other in their careers, and had an easy, affectionate relationship. Yet their sex life had never been good. At best, intercourse frequency was once a week. Joe would initiate in a clumsy, goal-oriented manner and he ejaculated early. Occasionally, Gail would be orgasmic, but this was rare, more a pleasant surprise than an integral part of sexual expression.

Joe went out of town for a six-week managerial training program and, during the first week, was seduced by one of the trainers. It was a most amazing sexual five weeks. Joe was introduced to oral sex, which increased his receptivity to penile stimulation and facilitated development of ejaculatory control. The trainer taught Joe how to stimulate a woman and he became aware that it was normal and expected for a woman to be orgasmic. When he returned home, he had to decide how to convey his newfound sexual interest and competence.

Joe chose not to reveal details, but he did tell Gail that he had a desire to make their sexual relationship more satisfying. Gail surmised he'd had an affair, but chose not to pursue the issue. She was receptive to his interest and was pleased by his new sexual comfort and skill. Within five months, they developed a satisfying couple sexual style. Joe was no longer looking back on the affair, but was enjoying a creative and playful sexual relationship with his wife. Gail was more responsive and orgasmic than ever before. With the help of his learning from the affair, marital sex was a functional part of their relationship, not a constant course of discontent. They were building a reservoir of shared sexual intimacy. Their implicit agreement was not to discuss Joe's affair, which was an appropriate choice for them. However, Gail made it clear that her responsiveness was based on Joe's commitment to being loyal to her and not having a pattern of affairs.

John and Helen. John and Helen's experience with integrating their affair is particularly enlightening. They'd been married twenty-three years. Early in the marriage, while John was in the service, both had had brief affairs; these had never been discussed. Shortly after the marriage of their oldest son, John began an affair with a younger single woman at work. This affair continued on an intermittent basis over a three-year period, and caused a good deal of disruption in the marriage and for the adolescent children still living at home.

John felt that this was his last chance to make a significant change in his life. The affair involved much sexual variety and excitement. John was motivated by a need to reaffirm his vitality and gain a sense of control over his life. Throughout this period, he continued to care for Helen, although there was a good deal of hurt and anger between them. Helen was not a martyr, but chose not to force John to leave the house and marriage. She dealt with her feelings by discussing issues with friends, and putting more energy into her job. She continued active involvement in parenting and had a number of personal activities and projects that affirmed her sense of self-worth.

After John's affair had run its course, they spent three weeks at a quiet beach. There was no dramatic Hollywood reconciliation, but they did make a commitment to revitalize their marriage. Feelings of hurt, vulnerability, resentment, and disappointment did not just vanish. The healing and rebuilding process occurred over a year's period, and even now there are scars and sensitive areas. Helen resented having to be the prime parent during those years and felt that John had taken her for granted and treated their marital bond in a disrespectful manner.

This marriage had enough strength to weather the storm and turmoil of an affair. John wonders if he would have had the emotional strength to maintain the marriage if the shoe had been on the other foot and it was Helen who'd had the affair. In the same way that there are seasons in a person's life, there are seasons in a marriage. John and Helen had a four-year winter, but with a renewed sense of commitment to their couple bond and a willingness to deal with their range of feelings, the relationship again bloomed.

PREVENTION OF AFFAIRS

Most prevention advice is simplistic and moralistic. Extra-marital sex is viewed as an evil to be prevented at all costs. This advice ignores the realities, opportunities, and complexities of extramarital sexuality in contemporary America. Each marriage is different, and interest in and opportunity for an extramarital affair has to be understood in the context of the marriage itself, the particular circumstances, and the individual involved.

In an ideal scenario, early in the marriage—and even before marriage—the couple would have a frank discussion about the role of marital sexuality, and share their thoughts and feelings about extramarital affairs. This is seldom done and the consequence is that it's not unusual for a couple to be sitting in a therapist's office dealing with the crisis of a discovered affair. It's not surprising since each person has had a different implicit assumption about affairs. Typically, the woman's assumption is that there will not be any affairs, and she will feel particularly vulnerable if it was she who has had the affair. The man's assumption is that he can have brief or discreet affairs—no harm is done if it "doesn't mean anything." He's surprised and shaken by the crisis caused by the affair.

A good guideline is that the better the marriage and marital sex, the more reason to decide against having an extramarital affair. It is too disruptive and draining, not worth putting a satisfying relationship under stress. Prevention is the most cost-efficient strategy.

Perhaps the best prevention technique is to have a clear understanding about the type of affair each partner is most vulnerable to and how to avoid falling into an affair. For example, women who are friendly and touchy are vulnerable to turning a male friendship into a sexual affair. A coping strategy would be for the husband to meet the men she works with or serves on committees with. She would state that she enjoys talking and being with friends, but has strong feelings of marital loyalty. For men who travel a lot or are in high-opportunity-for-affairs jobs—salesmen, police officers, or teachers—it is important to have a safe agenda such as working out, reading or writing, calling home, bringing a project or hobby to work on while on the road. Secrecy provides a fertile breeding ground for affairs. Spouses should commit to talk out a high-risk situation rather than feeling embarrassed or guilty and keeping it to themselves.

Another technique is to agree to tell your spouse that you are considering having an affair before acting on it. In movies, novels, and especially soap operas, people are swept away by uncontrollable urges. Our suggestion would not make good media, but it does make for a more resilient trust bond in a marriage. Your partner cannot force or coerce you to remain faithful. The sense of respect for your spouse should be strong enough that you keep your agreement to talk to him before acting on an affair. It will be a stressful and confrontative talk, but it will force each partner to examine how an affair will impact their life. It will also promote discussion of the risks of sexually transmitted disease and pregnancy, and the threat to the couple's marital and sexual relationship.

A different level of prevention occurs after an extramarital affair, when the choice is to revitalize the marriage. You need to discuss the meaning of the affair, and more important, how you can deal with it so that it does not burden the marital bond. The element most disrupted by an extramarital affair is trust. If the marriage is to be revitalized, you need to restore trust by making a clear agreement concerning future affairs. Most couples choose abstinence from affairs and put their energy into rebuilding the intimacy bond.

The extramarital affair need not become a "hot" supersensitive topic. Avoid the extremes of denial or obsessive focus. Life, sex, and marriage are meant to be lived in the present, not controlled by memories or grudges from the past. If an affair has occurred, learn from it. What was being communicated by the affair and what do you have to attend to in your lives and the marriage? The best prevention technique is to keep the marital bond of respect, trust, and intimacy strong and vital.

In writing this chapter and discussing these examples, we are not encouraging couples to experiment with extramarital affairs, and we are certainly not saying that what every marriage needs is an affair to rewaken emotional and sexual feelings. In our marriage, we have chosen—and it has been a conscious and discussed choice—not to have extramarital affairs. That decision comes from our awareness that trust and intimacy would be disrupted, although we do not believe it would be destroyed, by an affair.

OUR PERSONAL MARITAL AGREEMENT

We were proud that we discussed a number of issues before marrying. We reached agreements about contraception and planning children, where we would live, careers, sexuality, money, and dealing with in-laws. A notable area we did not discuss was extramarital affairs. In retrospect, we had the typical anxieties and inhibitions of other young couples. As our relationship progressed, we had more open conversations about sexuality, making requests, and trying to improve the quality of our marital sex. We studiously avoided any discussion of extramarital affairs.

The topic came up in serendipitous fashion. A male teaching assistant had a female student who was flunking. She approached the teaching assistant and offered to do anything he wanted Saturday night if she could only pass the course. The teaching assistant was both ethical and "up-tight," and told her that what she needed to do Saturday night was stay home and study. This story was greeted with great laughter, but afterward Emily asked Barry what he would do if a young woman approached him similarly. Barry tried his best to avoid dealing with the question, but Emily insisted that she wanted to talk this out and understand his viewpoint and feelings. Barry assured her that if he ever had an affair it would be totally separate from the marriage and would just be a fun fling for excitement and variety. This was Barry's implicit assumption about extramarital affairs, but it sounded strange being made explicit. Emily was adamant that if Barry had an option to have affairs, then to maintain a sense of equity she would want the same option. She was not interested in a one-night stand or a quick fling, but would want a sense of involvement in an affair. Barry was upset, and said that this kind of affair would be a threat to their marriage. Emily replied that if they were going to have an agreement about affairs, it had to be an equitable one.

We agreed that neither of us would have an affair. The advantage of talking about the issue and making an explicit agreement is that things are clear. The disadvantage is that if one or both partners break the agreement they will need to control feelings of disappointment and anger, and can't say it wasn't a big deal or that they didn't know.

Our agreement has worked well for us. We weren't suspicious when one traveled or went to dinner or to a meeting with a friend of the opposite sex. This is how we've chosen to deal with the issue of extramarital affairs, but it does not mean it will be the right choice for you. Each couple needs to consider their situation, marriage, and values and choose what is in their best interest. This is *our* decision rather than the "right" one. We do not want to imply a "holier than thou" attitude.

CLOSING THOUGHTS

Couples engage in extramarital affairs for different reasons, and the affair can have both helpful and harmful effects on the marriage. The resolution of the affair and how it is dealt with varies greatly. There is no "one right way" to handle extramarital affairs. A variety of reactions is normal. The main theme of this chapter is that, contrary to social pronouncements, many married people do have extramarital affairs and these can be dealt with if the couple is motivated to do so. An extramarital affair strains the trust bond, but need not break it. If the marriage is going to be vital and satisfying, the couple has to put time and energy into rebuilding respect, trust, intimacy, and sexuality.

17

SEX IN SECOND MARRIAGES

Marriage is not easy. Remarriage means a commitment to create a satisfying and stable relationship free of the disappointment and pain of the first. Folk wisdom has it that "There is no gathering the rose without being pricked by the thorns." When you marry, you do so with the fervent hope that this marriage will be satisfying and enduring: "Love 'til the twelfth of never." For over 40 percent of couples, this hope becomes a statistic—a divorce statistic. The failure of your marriage doesn't mean *you* are a failure or that a second marriage would be unwise. Choosing to divorce can be a sign of psychological health and good judgment, so that judging yourself a failure because of divorce is not reasonable. You are not a failure as a person, as a sexual being, or as a partner for a second marriage.

There are many reasons for divorce, the foremost being that marriage was entered into for the wrong reasons and/or that you chose an inappropriate partner. Other causes may be that the couple was not ready for marital commitment, that children born too soon put too much stress on the relationship, or that as the partners matured they changed in ways to which the marital relationship could not adapt. Divorce might also follow as a reaction to an extramarital affair, or because a couple did not devote time and energy to their marriage and grew apart.

Just as each marriage is unique, so are the reasons for dissolving it.

The primary reason for the increased divorce rate is that divorce is now accepted as a viable alternative to a poor marriage. Previously, there were strong family, religious, and societal pressures to remain married even if the marriage was a disaster for the individuals and the children. These external "glues" kept marginal and unsatisfying marriages intact. In the 1990s, the marital bond needs to be stronger and more viable. There are better quality marriages than a generation ago. There is also more marital dissolution because marriages that survived a generation ago because of external supports and the stigma of divorce do not survive in the 1990s. But is that really a loss?

Be aware of the causes for the dissolution of your first marriage. This is not to punish yourself and consider the marriage a failure, but to learn and benefit from the experience. What your learn about yourself and what you value in a relationship will help you to choose a second marriage that will be satisfying and enduring. The great majority of both men and women remarry. Second marriages are happier and more sexually fulfilling. This will be true if you have learned from your first experience, choose better, and put more time and psychological energy into your second marriage.

Susan. Susan married at nineteen, bore two children, divorced at twenty-eight, and, after a series of relationships, was considering remarriage at thirty-four. From her first experience she learned that marriage was not an answer to other problems, such as a desire to leave home, or uncertainty about vocational goals. She knew she was capable of living independently, enjoyed mothering her two children, and realized that she did not have to be married in order to function personally, sexually, and financially. In reviewing the first marriage, Susan knew she did not want to marry another man who drank heavily and who spent more time with the boys than with his wife and family. Susan liked active men who were ambitious and did not want to stay in the same house and job all their lives. She wanted a man who was willing to be an involved stepfather and interested in starting a second family.

Her years after the divorce had been painful and isolated at times, yet were worthwhile in that she had assumed more responsibility and felt good about herself as a person. Although her relationships during these years had not been particularly rewarding, either from a sexual or emotional viewpoint, neither had she deceived herself into thinking otherwise. Susan wanted to be planful, choiceful, and assertive in organizing her life. If she remarried, she wanted a partner whom she respected, trusted, and with whom she could share emotional and sexual intimacy. She also wanted greater financial security as well as a father for her children, since her first husband rarely saw the children. But these were not the most important factors in the decision to marry Rick. In Rick she found a male who was aware of her emotional and sexual feelings and open to feedback and guidance, and the critical factor for her was that he was willing to commit the time and energy to develop a satisfying and secure marital bond.

Susan's second marriage was likely to be successful because of her awareness, her sense of personal responsibility, and her realization that she could choose whether or not to remarry. Although three of four women and six of seven divorced men eventually remarry (the percentage is slightly lower for widows and widowers and considerably lower for older people), the alternative not to remarry is viable. A person can have a successful life—including a sexually functional life—without marriage. The best reason to remarry is the desire to share your life with another person. Many people remarry because it is expected, for security, to have a parent for their children, or to avoid loneliness. These can be valid and important factors, but when they are prime motives it is more difficult to choose well and to achieve a satisfying marriage. Marrying for negative reasons or deficit needs makes it less likely that you will assess your new partner realistically and discuss values, goals, and whether you are a viable couple. When your motives are positive you are much more likely to choose well and to develop a successful second marriage.

The most important guideline in a second marriage is not to play the "comparison game." Start fresh with your new spouse. Nowhere is this truer than in the bedroom. Many people, especially males, believe the myth that they know all there is to know about sex because of experiences with their first spouse and/or other partners. Sexually, each person is unique. Be aware of and acknowledge your partner's uniqueness instead of depending on what "worked" with previous partners. Be open to new sexual scenarios and stimulation techniques, and establish a feedback system to share what is and what isn't sexually attractive and pleasurable. Developing a couple sexual style takes practice and feedback, but most of all requires an awareness of the necessity to do so.

Ed. Ed had a poor marriage of fifteen years duration, although for the first ten years one good aspect was their sexual relationship, which degenerated when fighting, disillusionment, and bitterness increased. The event that eventually ended the marriage was Ed's discovery of his wife's extramarital affair. Soon after the divorce, she married the man with whom she'd had the affair. Even though Ed himself had had several affairs during the marriage he felt inadequate and obsessively worried that he was sexually inferior to the other man.

Two years later, Ed married Ann, who had been divorced for three years. When Ann was assertive and made sexual requests, Ed felt threatened, became hostile, and told her that if she did not like his way of making love she could find someone else. Ann began to think of Ed as an insecure, chauvinistic male. She was doing what was recommended in self-help books and the women's group she attended, and was frustrated that her sexual requests weren't working and instead were causing a major rift in the marriage. This was particularly galling because her first husband had objected adamantly when she'd learned to stand up for her rights. Ed became angry and defensive when Ann said anything about sexual technique because of his insecurity.

Luckily, Ed and Ann were intelligent people, cared about each other, and had enough of a commitment that they sought marital therapy. The clinician helped them to see that bad experiences from their first marriages were interfering with the development of a satisfying sexual relationship. With Ed's defensiveness identified and reduced, and Ann stating clearly that she cared for him and wanted to make the sexual relationship good for *both* of them, they could make sexual requests and guide each other. No longer threatened and inhibited, Ed became more comfortable and competent as a lover. With her fear of negative evaluation reduced, Ann became more responsive sexually. Occasionally, as almost all couples, they would fall into their old traps of being defensive and frustrated. They identified present problems they needed to deal with, and let go of inappropriate fears or resentments from the past.

Even if a person has had thirty years of positive sexual experiences, he needs to come into a second marriage with an open, receptive attitude. Each partner brings both helpful and harmful sexual attitudes and skills to a second marriage. To be a sexually functional couple you have to learn together. You are a new couple who have to develop a unique marital and sexual style. It will probably take at least six months to develop a high quality, intimate, sexually expressive relationship. This attitude is relevant not only to sexual issues but also communication techniques, nondestructive arguments, satisfactory agreements, enjoyment of each other, and increased marital commitment.

After being hurt in a first marriage, it is impossible for some people to make themselves vulnerable and to risk becoming deeply and intimately involved.

Terri. Terri was forty-three years old and still suffering psychological scars from her first marriage. Hers was the classic example of a nurse who marries a young man entering medical school. She gave up her career plans and worked extra jobs so that he could afford to finish school and an extended residency program. He was completely absorbed in completing his training and building a practice. During these years, few of Terri's needs were met, and there was little time for the marital relationship to thrive. Most of their sexual contacts were of the "slam, bam, thank you ma'am" variety (professional people, including psychologists, fall into this trap too). While her husband grew intellectually and underwent tremendous professional and personal changes, Terri's personal and professional life stagnated. Her role was to support her husband financially and give him freedom to pursue his medical career.

When Terri decided that it was time to quit her job and start a family, her husband shocked her with the news that he was no longer in love with her. He refused to have a child to shore up their failing marriage, and asked for a divorce. Terri was devastated, felt used and depressed, and attempted suicide. The divorce was bitter, and her subsequent years as a divorcée further disillusioned and hardened Terri.

In her second marriage, Terri did learn from the mistakes of the first and chose a man who was considerate and caring, and who clearly loved her. He did not ask her to give up personal plans, friends, or job. They reached mutually satisfying agreements on how to organize career and couple activities. It was extremely difficult for Terri to risk being emotionally vulnerable in this marriage. She was embittered that at forty-three she felt too old to start having children, angry at having been used and discarded by her first husband, and unwilling to commit herself to an intimate relationship in which she would once again risk being rejected. Because of Terri's reluctance, her husband became less emotionally involved. Her second marriage was vastly superior to the first, yet both Terri and her husband felt cheated that it was not the intimate, emotionally satisfying relationship it could have been.

John. A very different outcome occurred with John who chose to take risks and make himself vulnerable in his second marriage. He too felt manipulated and devastated by his first marriage. He had married Janie, whom he'd known in high school, when she became pregnant the summer after graduation. She had family and psychological problems, and used their marriage as a way to feel loved and worthwhile.

John was in the service when he married and in Vietnam

when his son was born. By the time he returned home, his marriage was in dire straits. Janie had been unable to tolerate the stress of living alone with a baby and had moved in with another man. John persuaded her to return, and they spent three conflict-ridden years attempting to salvage their poorly thought out marriage. It ended in a bitter divorce. John felt that the alimony and child support payments were excessive. Because of ongoing financial conflicts, he did not have regular contact with his son, which depressed him and all but destroyed the father-son bond.

John liked the idea of being married and having children. Even though his first experience had been bitter, it did not disillusion him about the intimacy and security possible in marriage. Because of his poor financial situation, he had to move in with his parents and take a second job. It took him over two years to get back on his feet financially and psychologically.

A year and a half later, John began dating Kathy, a divorced woman. Their relationship developed slowly. John and Kathy discussed their emotional reactions to the divorce experience and what it would take for them to be a successful and stable couple. The idealistic, romantic feelings and illusions experienced at eighteen are not repeated the second time around, nor should they be. We as a culture are enthralled with the concept of romantic love, but romantic love is not a good basis for a satisfying and secure marriage. The emotional highs that accompany a dating relationship motivate the person to take risks and become involved. Unfortunately, couples are swept away by the wave of romantic love and never discuss personal strengths and weaknesses nor objectively examine their relationship. The advantage couples like John and Kathy have is that they're motivated to take a critical look at themselves and their relationship before committing to marriage. You lose romantic mystique, but through a realistic appraisal of yourself, your partner, and your situation, you gain a more intimate relationship with a greater likelihood of success.

Their marriage has been committed and intimate for over ten years. Parenting their eight-year-old daughter has been highly satisfying for John. The divorce and its aftermath were traumatic, but did not so scar him that he wasn't willing to risk again. John and Kathy have achieved one of the best second marriages—or for that matter, *any* marriage—we know of.

GUIDELINES FOR A SECOND MARRIAGE

An open attitude and willingness to learn—the old cliché "nothing ventured, nothing gained"—is crucial to a successful second marriage. Second marriages can be, and usually are, better than first marriages. They are most successful when the person has learned from the first experience, has chosen a second spouse more wisely, risks being vulnerable and puts energy into the relationship, and is committed to making this marriage successful. The couple needs to share sexual experiences, be spontaneous and experimental, and to be aware of and responsive to the partner's desires. It is helpful to state your intentions directly: "I want our marriage to be good and satisfying. I have a lot to learn about you and you have a lot to learn about me. If we share as a couple, it can be fun. I want to know what makes you feel good, what arouses you, and what you don't like. I have to unlearn things from my first marriage, and I bet you do, too. Let's not be afraid to try. I love you and want sex to nurture and energize our marital bond."

Two major functions of sex in marriage are to reinforce and energize the bond and deepen and reinforce intimacy. A couple who are sexually open and vulnerable will generalize these attitudes and feelings to other areas of the marriage. Feeling good about your sexual bond helps to ease the inevitable hassles and adjustments in other areas. Second marriages can be complicated, especially in the initial years. Issues involving stepchildren and in-laws make blended families complex and challenging. An intimate sexual relationship is a solid basis for the marriage and provides motivation to deal with these issues.

Bob and Gloria. One of Barry's most difficult cases involved a couple who were engaged in a power struggle concerning the role of sex in their marriage. Bob was convinced that sexual problems had wrecked his first marriage, and was determined that in his second sex would be uninhibited and exciting. He insisted that Gloria's sexual withholding was the problem. He'd read a number of sex books, attended sexuality workshops, and perceived himself as committed to the time and energy needed to make this marriage sexually satisfying. Gloria felt defensive about Bob's sexual focus, and insisted that sex alone would not make their marriage work. Her first marriage, like Bob's, had been a sexual disaster. Gloria attributed this to her husband's immaturity and denial of problems. She felt that the only issue Bob was willing to deal with was sexuality, that he ignored and avoided talking about other issues and problems. The power struggle centered on Bob's unwillingness to make any agreements about their marriage until the sexual relationship improved. Gloria was unwilling to talk about sex until Bob showed that he cared by taking her to visit friends and relatives, and discussing house purchases, decorating, and other issues affecting their blended family.

Power struggles are counterproductive. They serve to do nothing other than build resentment. In a power struggle, not losing or giving in becomes more important than working together to reach marital agreement. You become so caught up in the struggle that you forget what you originally wanted. You are fighting not to win, but to avoid losing. Bob's sexual preoccupation and Gloria's fear of not being respected and cared for caused them to be protective and stubborn. Barry saw each in five sessions of individual therapy, in order to reduce defensiveness and achieve awareness of how self-defeating their stances were. Bob had to recognize that there was more to marriage than sex. Gloria realized that Bob's reluctance to interact socially with her friends and relatives did not mean he didn't want to be seen with her, but reflected his anxiety that they wouldn't like him. He was afraid he'd be taken advantage of, emotionally or financially, in a marriage where he didn't feel sexually valued. With these issues clarified, they were able to give up the power struggle and move forward to develop a marital and sexual style.

A major barrier in second marriages is the "fear of a repeat" phenomenon. The spouse is afraid that a fight, a money problem, sexual dysfunction, or whatever bad experiences caused her first marriage to disintegrate will recur in this marriage. To prevent that, she avoids fights, does what the other wants sexually, and refuses to discuss hurtful experiences. This avoidance strategy is self-defeating. You have to deal with issues, instead of avoiding them. You can learn from the prior marriage, but cannot let past fears control your self-esteem and new marriage. Use your awareness as a positive resource. Develop a problem-solving approach in which you work together and have a productive way to deal with sensitive issues.

Mary and George. Mary's first marriage had many problems, but what contributed most to the divorce were fights over money. Her husband would become angry and physically abuse her. Mary felt incapable of handling money matters or angry fights.

While she was single again and responsible for money management, she learned to handle finances quite well. In her second marriage, she was afraid the money management and abusive fight pattern would repeat itself. To prevent this, she turned over money, bills, checkbook—all financial matters to George. She would acquiesce on every issue, doing anything to avoid an argument.

The marriage went reasonably well for the first two years. Then resentments began to build. George had to assume all financial responsibilities with no help. He was annoyed by Mary's weakness and fear of anything to do with money. He began losing respect for her, and it was not long before loving feelings also waned. Mary herself felt that George did not make good financial decisions and that she did not have enough money to run the household. Constantly trying to avoid arguments caused tension, resulting in headaches. Feelings of competence and confidence she'd developed while single were dissipating.

The lack of working together as a couple spilled over to the sexual area. Their sex life became routine and boring, and neither felt a sense of sharing. Resentment from other areas indirectly affects the couple's sexual relationship. This cycle built on itself and became increasingly erosive.

Avoiding issues that caused problems in the first marriage is unrealistic. A more productive strategy is to be aware of and to monitor the sensitive area. For example, Mary might have told George that money problems and fights were a trap for her, that they needed to work out a satisfactory set of agreements about financial matters. They might develop a plan assigning each specific money management responsibilities, and set a weekly time to discuss how the system was working. She would be encouraged to express any bad feelings in a nondestructive manner, and to engage in problem-solving to reach agreements instead of destructive, painful fights. After a disagreement, there would be time set aside the next day to discuss how it was handled, especially whether Mary found it worthwhile to air the bad feelings and to be sure the resolution was acceptable. In marriage, as in other areas of life, a preventive approach is the most economical and helpful. Developing a system to deal with difficult issues and setting aside time to discuss how you're handling them is an excellent strategy for dealing with the "avoidance trap."

CLOSING THOUGHTS

Second marriages face a myriad of complex practical and emotional issues, including dealing with stepchildren, child support payments, friends and relatives from the past marriage, feelings of resentment and/or competition regarding the previous spouse, and the functioning of the blended family. Be aware of these issues and be willing to devote time and psychological energy to them.

Whole books have been written on blended families (stepfamilies). It's important to accept that this family system is different from, and more complex than, the traditional nuclear family. These complexities need to be dealt with instead of pretending that everyone loves each other and that this is the best possible outcome for all concerned. In complex situations, there are always ambivalent feelings. Some issues will not be resolved in a successful manner—sometimes a child does not like his stepparent or an ex-spouse continues to be angry and resentful. The best way to deal with these inevitable conflicts and disappointments is to continue to strengthen the primary relationship in the family, your husband-wife bond. Strive to achiever positive changes and accept that some problems cannot be remedied. Remember, ''The Waltons'' made great TV, but no family, nuclear or blended, lives up to that ideal.

We would like to reiterate two themes. Learning from the mistakes and problems of the first marriage greatly increases the probability that you will choose better and that the second marriage will be more intimate and satisfying. Secondly, adopting an open attitude that stresses the need to learn about each other, argue constructively, reach satisfactory agreements, have fun, and develop your sexual style insures that this marriage will be fulfilling and secure.

18
COPING WITH STRESS AND ILLNESS

Our theme throughout the book has been positive: your marital and sexual relationship can be satisfying rather than stagnating and problematic. You can continue to learn and grow as individuals and as a couple, which will result in greater intimacy and satisfaction.

In this chapter we would like to emphasize a concept that has been given only passing attention by most marriage books. The sign of a good marriage is not that the couple are happy when external events are going well and there are few problems. A worthwhile, solid marriage is demonstrated by the couple's ability to support each other through crises and losses and to cope with problems as they arise. Some couples naïvely hope that if they follow our guidelines they will have no difficulties in their marriage. Nothing could be further from the truth. The more you understand your marital and sexual relationship, the better you can deal with problems and prevent yourself from falling into the most common traps.

You will be confronted with difficult situations. They happen in our lives and marriage, and will in yours, and may include a parent becoming disabled and your needing to help care for him, your being unemployed for six months, a child with diabetes who needs careful monitoring, your best friends getting divorced, your spouse having colon cancer, an adolescent child becoming pregnant, a career risk not working, a prostate operation that results in retrograde ejaculation, a life-threatening accident to a child, a college degree or training program that doesn't lead to a suitable job, an extramarital affair that promotes feelings of distrust and anger, a job change that necessitates a geographic move and causes family disruption. These events can and do happen in almost every marriage. Some can be prevented, many cannot.

One test of the viability of a marriage is your willingness to deal with painful situations and experiences. An essential difference between those who maintain psychological well-being and psychologically troubled people is not the number of good things that happen, but their ability to cope with the bad ones. Coping with difficulties means accepting their reality and attempting to regain equilibrium without major psychological scars. The best way to deal with a crisis is to see it as an opportunity for learning. If you cope successfully, your trust in each other will be stronger.

Psychologists have developed a theory of how people cope with a bad experience. In the first stage there is denial or rejection of the event (it can't really be happening). This is followed by a sense of anger (why the hell did this happen to me?), and then a feeling of despair and depression (this is too terrible; I can't deal with it; I'll never be able to accept it). In the final stage of integration, the process reaches a resolution (it was a terrible experience, but I've dealt with it and can go on with my life). You accept the incident and see yourself as an active survivor rather than a passive victim. Be aware of this process, stay with it, don't repress feelings. You will cope and survive. One of our favorite one-liners is "Living well is the best revenge." As you reestablish your life and marriage, look back on the stress and trauma and acknowledge that you survived and have reassumed control of your life. Life is meant to be lived in the present, planning for and anticipating the future. It is not meant to be controlled by trauma and resentment from the past.

Jim and Tina. Jim and Tina, a couple in their early forties, were feeling satisfied with life. They'd been married seventeen years, had a son fourteen and a daughter twelve. Jim was an airplane mechanic and Tina an advertising account executive. With two good incomes they lived well, traveled, and engaged in a variety of couple and family activities. They had a good marriage and a satisfying sexual relationship.

The initial stress came from Tina discovering a lump during a monthly breast self-examination. Her battle with cancer was to be a prolonged one that was physically, financially, and psychologically draining for her, the marriage, and the family. She underwent a mastectomy and extensive chemotherapy. During this time the children were going through adolescence, which is stressful for most couples. Jim was afraid of being a widower with two teenagers, and his fear made it more difficult to listen to and emotionally support Tina during the cancer treatments. Unlike crises described in books and popular magazine articles, which are intense but limited to hours or days, theirs extended over a five-year period. Tina won her battle with cancer; but, as with all diseases in remission, fears of recurrence are present. Interestingly, they sought marital therapy not during the height of the crisis, but waited until a year had passed (We strongly recommend that couples going through a stressful period seek professional help *at the time*.) Both Jim and Tina felt emotionally drained and their marriage was exhausted. They had sex less than once a month and it was not satisfying.

They finally stopped avoiding the situation, confronted it, and were motivated to begin dealing with issues. The rebuilding process was a slow one with several missteps and frustrating experiences, yet they maintained commitment and trust in their marital bond. One of the worst traps was to look back to earlier times, when things seemed natural and simple. Revitalizing their marriage was difficult because they had to overcome inertia, and they found it hard to set aside couple time. Jim and Tina had to accept that they were not a young, energetic couple filled with the ecstasy of romantic love, but a middle-aged couple who had shared and coped with a good deal of stress and needed time to reenergize themselves. They couldn't go back to easier times; they had to persevere in the task of recovering from a prolonged crisis and building a satisfying future.

June and Paul. Dealing with loss puts special stress on a marriage. Perhaps the worst loss is the death of a child. There is no "right" way to make the feelings less intense. It is a most painful experience, and will have a profound effect on you, the marriage, and sexuality. Barry saw June and Paul when their son, Ronald, was still in a coma. This eight-year-old boy had suffered severe injuries in a car accident. Even if he had lived, the damage to his brain would have left him profoundly handicapped physically and intellectually. Sessions would sometimes include the entire family, other times just the couple. Individual sessions were scheduled with June who had been driving the car.

The first task was to help them accept the reality of Ronald's impending death. Paul wanted to consult the world's greatest brain surgeon instead of allowing himself to cry and to begin mourning his only son. Ronald's sisters expressed their feelings of grief and sadness better than the parents. At the funeral, the minister's sensitive sermon and their friends' genuine sorrow provided support for the family.

In the ensuing months, Paul and June experienced a range of emotions from guilt and anger to listlessness and depression. Slowly they became reinvolved in their lives and experienced times of joy and excitement. They attended to the needs of their daughters, but did not put pressure on them to compensate for the loss of Ronald. They would always consider themselves the parents of three children, one of whom had been tragically killed at age eight. The stress and sadness of that experience did not destroy their marital bond because June and Paul supported each other through the grieving process. The sense of trust and coupleness helped them, and their children, to begin living once again in the present.

STRESSES OF PARENTING

One of the major joys in marriage is parenting children. It is also one of the major stresses. This is true of all marriages. An ill child, an acting-out or rejecting adolescent, can strain the best of marital bonds.

There are two guidelines to understand and cope with the stresses of parenting. The first is to view the problem in terms of the family system rather than to blame yourself or the child, to feel guilty, or give up. The second is to remember that you are first a person, then a spouse, and then a parent. In the long run you will be a better parent if you do not sacrifice your sense of self and marital bond.

Parenting is a crucial role that requires a large and consistent expenditure of time and psychological energy. Be aware of the joys and satisfactions of parenting. Develop individual and couple activities to provide a break and reinforcement for parenting. The first step is to acknowledge that problems exist rather than to pretend that there are none. Don't feel you are a bad person or a bad mother if you find parenting stressful.

The stress that comes from having a baby can be overwhelming. The fact that a baby is so helpless and needy, combined with your lack of skill and worry that you are not the "perfect" caretaker, is draining. When our youngest son was ten days old he stopped breathing. Luckily, our next door neighbor was an emergency room nurse and revived him. We didn't go back to sleeping through the night for several weeks after that incident. During that period, sex was the furthest thing from our minds.

As the child becomes a toddler, you worry that he may hurt himself exploring the world. Many women find the preschool years particularly stressful. You feel you don't have a second to yourself. There is always the possibility of tears or problems. Unless you make specific arrangements and plans, the only time you have to be sexual is late at night when the children are asleep. Late night sex when you're exhausted is not likely to be a good time for creative, playful sexuality.

Parents look forward to having more time when children enter school, and are surprised to discover new stress in dealing with teachers, other parents, PTA, etc. Others are sharing the caretaking of your child, but this requires sharing control of the child as well as assuming additional responsibilities. You have to decide who will go to parent-teacher meetings, monitor homework, drive car pools. If both parents work, who assumes child care during school holidays, snow days, or illness? Unless you have had to deal with these realities, it is hard to describe how difficult and burdensome they can be.

The years from seven to eleven are called the ''golden years of childhood.'' They were among our favorite years of parenting, but this doesn't mean they are stress-free. Trouble with school performance, a difficult adjustment to a friend's moving away, problems with a sibling or neighbor, illness or accident, embarrassment over beginning menstruation or wet dreams—the parent must deal seriously with all these concerns rather than treating them lightly or shrugging them off as unimportant childhood problems. These things matter to your child, and it matters that you be a caring and responsive parent. Throughout childhood, but especially at this age, it is important to be an ''askable parent.'' The child needs to know she can come to you with questions and issues regarding psychological and sexual, as well as practical and educational matters. A particular problem for children is their feeling that when something bad happens they need to keep it secret rather than to consult the parent as a resource and helper. Parents need to both nurture and discipline.

Junior high school and early adolescent years can be particularly stressful. For many, this is the beginning of experimentation—or at least flirtation—with smoking, drinking, drugs, and sexuality. There is a real struggle between peer group and family influence. Children who were good students in elementary school might find the transition to junior high disruptive. Some students experience a dramatic drop in academic motivation, and adopt the stance of alienated adolescent. The type of discipline and rewards that were successful a year before no longer work. The parent who was a ''Super Mom'' or ''Super Dad'' two years ago is now a subject of derision as not being ''with it.''

Are the adolescent years as bad as some say? Certainly not for all adolescents and parents. However, thirteen to sixteen is the most unhappy time in a person's life and for a significant number of parents of adolescents it's a time of stress on their marriage. The parents' major motivation is fear—of pregnancy, drinking and driving, peer pressure, sexually transmitted diseases and AIDS, drugs, self-destructive behavior. One of our children was an acting-out adolescent, and we found it very stressful. Our coping techniques were going for walks and going out to eat (a positive side effect was that we developed a love of ethnic food). Emily remembers Barry telling her, "We will survive this as individuals and as a couple." There were times when she wondered. In fact, all of us survived. Life gets better after adolescence, not only for the adolescent but for the couple, too.

Parenting does not end when the child becomes an eighteen-year-old young adult. It doesn't even end when the person is a twenty-five-year-old adult, even if marriage with children of her own. Parenting will become less stressful as you take more of a consultant role and feel less burdened by responsibilities. That is not always true, especially if you are paying for a child's training program, or college, or helping finance a house. Hopefully, you will experience satisfaction from these endeavors.

Much has been written about the syndrome "empty nest". The majority of couples report this as a time of increased personal freedom, couple intimacy, and more frequent and higher quality sex. Couples enjoy the process of parenting, but it's exciting to return to being a couple again and to experience a life of reduced stress and responsibility.

CHANGING OLD ATTITUDES AND HABITS

Many couples look at their marriages and feel so strongly tied to old attitudes and habits that they believe there is no way to change. The only way out seems to be divorce and/or an affair. In taking this viewpoint, you negate your partner's ability to change and don't trust that you can influence her. We knew a man who for twenty-two years bristled because his wife would not leave a party early, afraid that she would hurt the hostess's feelings. He felt he could do nothing about this behavior. He did not believe she would listen to a direct request for change, and felt that they would never be able to reach a mutually agreeable solution. It is stressful and depressing to feel you are caught in an unsatisfying, unchangeable pattern. A major trap in ongoing marriages is losing trust in your ability to make requests, negotiate, and reach an agreement that will meet your needs and the needs of the marriage. In a caring relationship, there is always room for change. When a friend talked to the wife and made her aware of her husband's frustration, she was quite willing to change and leave parties when he was ready. She had not realized he really was bothered by this behavior. The husband was shocked and very pleased. His wife was irritated that he'd had to send an emissary rather than talking to her directly.

Marriage should be a reinforcing process, in which you bring out the best in each other. For many couples, the spouse is their best friend, someone to trust, who will be honest and not disparaging. As the TV commercials say, it's bad if "even your best friend won't tell you."

We all have idiosyncracies that were acceptable—and, at times, funny—when we were younger. As we age, these traits can become exaggerated, or we develop habits that are unacceptable to our spouse and, perhaps, to other people. A spouse or best friend has every right to make us aware of this and to have enough influence that we attend to the complaint. The spouse who no longer controls his drinking, complains constantly about past job or financial setbacks, has a pattern of watching TV and ignoring family members, gains weight and does not attend to personal appearance, does not keep up couple friendships, or becomes so involved in community and political affairs that marital and family needs are ignored—creates stress and needs to be confronted. In courting and early marriage, your spouse had a good deal of influence because you wanted him to love and care about you. There is no reason for this influence to lessen because you've been married for a number of years. In fact, in good marriages, positive influence increases, and there is a greater openness to sharing all aspects of your life, including stresses and problems. Value the caring of your spouse and be open to her requests and influence.

Jon and Judy. Jon and Judy had a big party to celebrate their silver—twenty-fifth—anniversary. Judy was feeling satisfied with her life. She enjoyed more freedom now that there were no children living at home, and savored a sense of accomplishment from her job. She was taken aback when, a week after the party, Jon expressed a need to discuss a major problem. He was feeling frustrated, he explained, with his job and their life. Years ago, they had moved to a suburban area because they wanted a larger home and better schools. They felt it was an excellent environment in which to raise children. Now, Jon wanted to move to a townhouse in the city, both to reduce his commuting time and to take advantage of the restaurants and cultural offerings of the city. He also wanted to resign his job and to set up his own consulting firm so that he could implement his creative ideas. Judy was distressed because she identified with her home and neighborhood. Her job was in a shopping center less than a mile away.

A key element in marriage is the ability to be aware of individual needs and feelings, and Jon had done that very well. Clear and direct communication is important in marriage, but does not automatically make things all right. It took a great deal of discussion and negotiation on both the practical and psychological aspects of the decision before a mutually acceptable agreement was reached.

They moved to a townhouse in an area of the city that Judy enjoyed. She became involved in the new community but retained her job in the suburbs and bought a sports car she could enjoy commuting in. Jon kept a consulting position with his employer rather than starting completely on his own. These decisions reflect the practical components of the agreement. More important was their discussion of the psychological and relationship meanings of the change. Instead of allowing their good marriage to "go along as is," they made a renewed commitment to individual and couple growth. Jon had seen a number of friends become dissatisfied with their jobs, marriages, and sex lives. He saw them drinking too much, having heart attacks, starting affairs with twenty-five-year-old secretaries, and becoming cynical and depressed. He was determined that this would not happen to him. Judy was able to hear Jon's feelings, fears, and requests without becoming afraid or defensive. One of their marital strengths was a sense of trust and equity. This allowed Judy to discuss her desires, feelings, and anxieties frankly without fearing that she would give in to Jon out of weakness, or agree to something she couldn't live with. Judy knew what was important to her, and was able to state that to Jon. From a position of awareness and caring for the other, they discussed feelings and negotiated an agreement both could live with.

A key element of satisfying marriage is openness to change and growth. It has been assumed that marriage is characterized by stability, but although stability and security are important, so are change and growth. People's lives, jobs, and parenting roles experience periods of transition. This is reflected in sexual functioning. The basis of creative sexual expression is an integration of the familiar and the secure (what you've learned brings sexual pleasure to you) and the immediate moods, techniques, and desires you bring to each sexual encounter. Your sexual relationship will be more alive and vital because of your having experienced changes. Marital trust and security provides the solid basis that allows you to be spontaneous and experimental, to take risks to be sexually creative.

SEXUAL STRESS

One of the best-kept secrets in this field is that the great majority of couples undergo a period of sexual stress sometime in their marriage. It can be caused by a specific sexual problem, such as erectile dysfunction, inhibited sexual desire, or painful intercourse; by a marital or family problem such as financial stress, a child in trouble, or a falling-out with another couple; by an individual problem such as depression, overwork, a strained back; or by an unexplained sense of malaise. How can a couple cope with sexual stress? Admit that this period is not a happy one for you, but do not overreact. Continue to accept your partner and maintain affectional and sexual contact. Even when sex is in remission, love, caring, and sensuality need to be expressed. This atmosphere of acceptance without blame allows a smoother return to satisfying sex as the issue is dealt with and the stress dissipates.

Some bemoan the loss of ecstasy in marital sex. If you examine ecstasy, you find it is most prevalent in premarital and extramarital affairs. The elements that comprise it are novelty, overcoming frustrations and barriers in order to be with the partner, sense of unpredictability, desire to be accepted and/or win the partner, and a sense of illicitness. This adventuresome, romantic notion of love is by definition fragile and temporary. It can and should be replaced by a mature sense of caring, security, respect, trust, and emotional intimacy. This provides a stable basis for a satisfying marriage and marital sex which will help you through the inevitable stresses human beings encounter.

EPILOGUE

This completes a four-book sequence. The first book was *Sexual Awareness: Enhancing Sexual Pleasure,* which focused on specific exercises to improve sexual comfort and pleasure. *Male Sexual Awareness: Increasing Sexual Satisfaction* and *Female Sexual Awareness: Achieving Sexual Fulfillment* focused on changing attitudes, behavior, and emotional responsiveness. We see this book as the crown jewel of the series. Optimal sexual functioning integrates emotional intimacy and sexual expression in the context of a secure marital bond.

Both women and men need to be comfortable and skilled at sexual initiation, sharing feelings, nondemand pleasuring, multiple stimulation, being orgasmic, and feeling close and bonded. Sex is more than genitals, intercourse, and orgasm. Sexuality is a positive, integral component in a marriage. It serves as a shared pleasure, a way to maintain and reinforce intimacy, and a tension reducer. When sexuality is doing well in marriage it is perhaps 15-20 percent, its primary function being to energize the marital bond.

We have tried to present models and guidelines to help couples increase their marital and sexual satisfaction. Each couple develops their unique marital and sexual style. We urge you to value your marriage and devote consistent time and psychological energy to nurture the marital bond, but we are not romantic idealists. There are no perfect jobs, no perfect children, no perfect houses, and no perfect marriages. Romantic images of marriage need to be replaced by mature intimacy. The marital bond of respect and trust enables you to accept your spouse and marriage for its strengths and joys as well as its weaknesses and problems. Marriage and marital sex are not static, both are a process of development and growth. Marriage works best when it is based on a positive influence model. Being married brings out the best in you as a person.

Sexuality can be a satisfying part of life and marriage. The essence of sexuality is giving and receiving touching and pleasure. Sexuality functions best in the context of a respectful, trusting, emotionally intimate marriage based on a sense of equity between a woman and a man. You owe it to yourself, spouse, and family to devote the time and psychological energy to make your marriage and marital sex satisfying and stable.

APPENDIX I
CHOOSING A THERAPIST

As we stated from the outset, this was not meant to be a do-it-yourself therapy book. Couples are sometimes reluctant to consult a professional therapist, feeling that to do so is a sign of "craziness," inadequacy, or that their marriage is in dire straits. We believe seeking professional help is a sign of psychological strength. Entering marital or sex therapy means that you realize there is a problem and that you've made a commitment to marital and sexual growth.

The mental health field is confusing. Marital and sex therapy is a subspeciality clinical skill. It is offered by several groups of professionals including psychologists, social workers, marriage therapists, psychiatrists, sex therapists, and pastoral counselors. The background of the practitioner is of less importance than her competency in dealing with your specific problem.

Many people have health insurance that provides coverage for mental health and thus they can afford the services of a private practitioner. Those who do not have either financial resources or insurance could consider a city or county mental health clinic, a university or medical-school mental health outpatient clinic, or a family services center. Clinics usually have a sliding fee scale— that is, the fee is based on your ability to pay.

In choosing a therapist be assertive in asking about his credentials and areas of expertise as well as his fees. Ask the clinician what percentage of her clients stay married, how long the therapy can be expected to last, and whether there is a specific focus on sexual dysfunction or problem-solving techniques. A competent therapist will be open to discussing this. Be especially diligent in questioning credentials such as university degrees and licensing, of people who call themselves personal counselors, marriage counselors, or sex counselors, since there are poorly qualified persons—and some outright quacks—in any field.

One of the best resources for obtaining a referral to a marital or sex therapist is to call a local professional organization such as a psychological association, mental health association, or mental health clinic. You can ask for a referral from a family physician, minister, or friend who has information on a therapist's areas of competence.

If you have a problem that principally concerns marriage or family issues, you could write the American Association for Marriage and Family Therapy, 1717 K Street, N. W., Room 407, Washington, D.C. 20006, for a list of certified marriage and family therapists in your area. If you are specifically interested in sex therapy, you can write the American Association of Sex Educators, Counselors, and Therapists, Suite 1717, 435 N. Michigan Avenue, Chicago, Ill. 60611 for a list of certified sex therapists in your area.

Feel free to talk with two or three therapists before deciding on one with whom to work. Be aware of how comfortable you feel with the therapist, the degree of rapport, and whether the therapist's assessment of the problem and approach to treatment make sense to you. Once you begin therapy, give it a chance to be helpful. There are few "miracle cures." Change requires commitment and is a gradual and often difficult process. The role of the therapist is that of consultant rather than decision-maker for you. Marital and sex therapy requires effort, both in the session and at home. Therapy can help change attitudes, feelings, and behavior, and make your marital and sexual life more satisfying.

APPENDIX II
BOOKS FOR FURTHER READING

Andry, Andrew, and Steve Schepp. *How Babies Are Made*. Boston: Little, Brown, 1984.

Barbach, Lonnie, and Linda Levine. *Shared Intimacies*. New York: Bantam Books, 1980.

Beck, Aaron. *Love is Never Enough*. New York: Harper and Row, 1988.

Bing, Elizabeth, and Libby Coleman. *Making Love During Pregnancy*. New York: Bantam Books, 1983.

Blumstein, Philip, and Pepper Schwartz. *American Couples*. New York: William Morrow, 1983.

Boston Women's Health Book Collective. *The New Our Bodies, Ourselves*. New York: Simon and Schuster, 1984.

Butler, Robert, and Myrna Lewis. *Love and Sex After Forty*. New York: Harper and Row, 1986.

Calderone, Mary, and Eric Johnson. *The Family Book About Sexuality*. New York: Harper and Row, 1989.

Downing, George. *The Massage Book*. New York: Random House, 1972.

Gordon, Sol. *Why Love is Not Enough*. Boston: Bob Adams, 1988.

Gordon, Sol, and Judith Gordon. *Raising a Child Conservatively in a Sexually Permissive World*. New York: Simon and Schuster, 1983.

Gottman, John, Cliff Notarius, Jonnie Gonso, and Howard Makkman. *A Couple's Guide to Communication*. Champaign, Illinois: Research Press, 1976.

Heiman, Julia, and Joseph LoPiccolo. *Becoming Orgasmic*. New York: Prentice Hall, 1988.

Lehner, Harriet. *The Dance of Intimacy*. New York: Harper and Row, 1989.

Lehner, Harriet. *The Dance of Anger*. New York: Harper and Row, 1985.

Levine, Linda, and Lonnie Barbach. *The Intimate Male*. New York: Doubleday, 1983.

Maltz, Wendy, and Beverly Holman. *Incest and Sexuality*. Lexington, Massachusetts: Lexington Books, 1987.

Masters, William, Virginia Johnson, and Robert Kolodny. *Masters and Johnson on Sex and Human Loving*. Boston: Little, Brown, 1986.

McCarthy, Barry. *Male Sexual Awareness*. New York: Carroll and Graf, 1988.

McCarthy, Barry, and Emily McCarthy. *Sexual Awareness*. New York: Carroll and Graf, 1984.

McCarthy, Barry, and Emily McCarthy. *Female Sexual Awareness*. New York, Carroll and Graf, 1989.

Nowinski, Joseph. *A Lifelong Love Affair*. New York: Dodd, Mead, 1988.

Sarrel, Lorna, and Philip Sarrel. *Sexual Turning Points*. New York: MacMillan, 1984.

Trafford, Abigail. *Crazy Time: Surviving Divorce*. New York: Bantam, 1982.

Zilbergeld, Bernie. *Male Sexuality*. New York: Bantam Books, 1978.

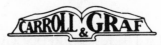

FINE WORKS OF NON-FICTION AVAILABLE IN QUALITY PAPERBACK EDITIONS FROM CARROLL & GRAF

☐ Anderson, Nancy/WORK WITH PASSION	$8.95
☐ Arlett, Robert/THE PIZZA GOURMET	$10.95
☐ Asprey, Robert/THE PANTHER'S FEAST	$9.95
☐ Bedford, Sybille/ALDOUS HUXLEY	$14.95
☐ Berton, Pierre/KLONDIKE FEVER	$10.95
☐ Blake, Robert/DISRAELI	$14.50
☐ Blanch, Lesley/PIERRE LOTI	$10.95
☐ Blanch, Lesley/THE WILDER SHORES OF LOVE	$8.95
☐ Buchan, John/PILGRIM'S WAY	$10.95
☐ Carr, John Dickson/THE LIFE OF SIR ARTHUR CONAN DOYLE	$8.95
☐ Carr, Virginia Spencer/THE LONELY HUNTER: A BIOGRAPHY OF CARSON McCULLERS	$12.95
☐ Cherry-Garrard/THE WORST JOURNEY IN THE WORLD	$13.95
☐ Conot, Robert/JUSTICE AT NUREMBURG	$11.95
☐ Cooper, Duff/OLD MEN FORGET	$10.95
☐ Cooper, Lady Diana/AUTOBIOGRAPHY	$13.95
☐ De Jonge, Alex/THE LIFE AND TIMES OF GRIGORII RASPUTIN	$10.95
☐ Edwards, Anne/SONYA: THE LIFE OF COUNTESS TOLSTOY	$8.95
☐ Elkington, John/THE GENE FACTORY	$8.95
☐ Farson, Negley/THE WAY OF A TRANSGRESSOR	$9.95
☐ Garbus, Martin/TRAITORS AND HEROES	$10.95
☐ Gill, Brendan/HERE AT THE NEW YORKER	$12.95
☐ Goldin, Stephen & Sky, Kathleen/THE BUSINESS OF BEING A WRITER	$8.95
☐ Golenbock, Peter/HOW TO WIN AT ROTISSERIE BASEBALL	$8.95
☐ Harris, A./SEXUAL EXERCISES FOR WOMEN	$8.95
☐ Haycraft, Howard (ed.)/THE ART OF THE MYSTERY STORY	$9.95
☐ Hook, Sidney/OUT OF STEP	$14.95
☐ Keating, H. R. F./CRIME & MYSTERY: THE 100 BEST BOOKS	$7.95
☐ Lansing, Alfred/ENDURANCE: SHACKLETON'S INCREDIBLE VOYAGE	$8.95
☐ Leech, Margaret/REVEILLE IN WASHINGTON	$11.95
☐ Lifton, David S./BEST EVIDENCE	$11.95

☐ Madden, David and Bach, Peggy/REDISCOVERIES II **$9.95**
☐ McCarthy, Barry and Emily/FEMALE SEXUAL
AWARENESS **$9.95**
☐ McCarthy, Barry/MALE SEXUAL AWARENESS **$9.95**
☐ McCarthy, Barry & Emily/SEXUAL AWARENESS **$9.95**
☐ Mizener, Arthur/THE SADDEST STORY: A
BIOGRAPHY OF FORD MADOX FORD **$12.95**
☐ Morris, Charles/IRON DESTINIES, LOST
OPPORTUNITIES: THE POST-WAR ARMS
RACE **$13.95**
☐ Moorehead, Alan/THE RUSSIAN REVOLUTION **$10.95**
☐ Munthe, Alex/THE STORY OF SAN MICHELE **$8.95**
☐ O'Casey, Sean/AUTOBIOGRAPHIES I **$10.95**
☐ O'Casey, Sean/AUTOBIOGRAPHIES II **$10.95**
☐ Poncins, Gontran de/KABLOONA **$9.95**
☐ Pringle, David/SCIENCE FICTION: THE 100
BEST NOVELS **$7.95**
☐ Proust, Marcel/ON ART AND LITERATURE **$8.95**
☐ Richelson, Hildy & Stan/INCOME WITHOUT
TAXES **$9.95**
☐ Roy, Jules/THE BATTLE OF DIENBIENPHU **$8.95**
☐ Salisbury, Harrison/A JOURNEY FOR OUR TIMES **$10.95**
☐ Scott, Evelyn/ESCAPADE **$9.95**
☐ Sloan, Allan/THREE PLUS ONE EQUALS BILLIONS **$8.95**
☐ Stanway, Andrew/THE ART OF SENSUAL
LOVING **$15.95**
☐ Trench, Charles/THE ROAD TO KHARTOUM **$10.95**
☐ Werth, Alexander/RUSSIA AT WAR: 1941–1945 **$15.95**
☐ White, Jon Manchip/CORTES **$10.95**
☐ Wilson, Colin/THE MAMMOTH BOOK OF
TRUE CRIME **$8.95**
☐ Zuckmayer, Carl/A PART OF MYSELF **$9.95**

Available from fine bookstores everywhere or use this coupon for ordering.

Carroll & Graf Publishers, Inc., 260 Fifth Avenue, N.Y., N.Y. 10001

Please send me the books I have checked above. I am enclosing
$_____ (please add $1.00 per title to cover postage and
handling.) Send check or money order—no cash or C.O.D.'s
please. N.Y. residents please add 8¼% sales tax.

Mr/Mrs/Ms _____

Address _____

City _____ State/Zip _____
Please allow four to six weeks for delivery.